Top Tips in Urology

Top Tips in Urology

Edited by

John McLoughlin
MS, FRCSUrol
Consultant Urological Surgeon
West Suffolk Hospital
Bury St Edmunds, UK

Neil Burgess
MCh, FRCSUrol
Consultant Urological Surgeon
Norfolk and Norwich University
Hospital
Norwich, UK

Hanif Motiwala
FRCS (Edin), FRCS (Urol)
Consultant Urological Surgeon
Heatherwood and Wexham Park
Hospital
Slough, UK

Mark J. Speakman
MS, FRCS
Consultant Urological Surgeon
Musgrove Park Hospital
Taunton, UK

Andrew Doble
MS, FRCSUrol
Consultant Urological Surgeon
Addenbrooke's Hospital
Cambridge, UK

John D. Kelly
MD, FRCSUrol
Professor of Urology
Honorary Consultant Urological
Surgeon
University College Hospital
London, UK

SECOND EDITION

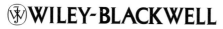

A John Wiley & Sons, Ltd., Publication

This edition first published 2013, © 2013 by John Wiley & Sons, Ltd

Wiley-Blackwell is an imprint of John Wiley & Sons, formed by the merger of Wiley's global Scientific, Technical and Medical business with Blackwell Publishing.

Registered Office
John Wiley & Sons, Ltd, The Atrium, Southern Gate, Chichester, West Sussex,
PO19 8SQ, UK

Editorial Offices
9600 Garsington Road, Oxford, OX4 2DQ, UK
The Atrium, Southern Gate, Chichester, West Sussex, PO19 8SQ, UK
111 River Street, Hoboken, NJ 07030-5774, USA

For details of our global editorial offices, for customer services and for information about how to apply for permission to reuse the copyright material in this book please see our website at www.wiley.com/wiley-blackwell.

Library of Congress Cataloging-in-Publication Data

Top tips in urology / edited by John McLoughlin ... [et al.]. – 2nd ed.
    p. ; cm.
  Includes bibliographical references and index.
  ISBN 978-0-470-67293-8 (pbk. : alk. paper)
  I. McLoughlin, J.
  [DNLM: 1. Urogenital System–surgery–Handbooks. 2. Surgical Procedures,
Operative–methods–Handbooks. WJ 39]
  616.6–dc23
                                            2012032719

A catalogue record for this book is available from the British Library.

Wiley also publishes its books in a variety of electronic formats. Some content that appears in print may not be available in electronic books.

Cover design by Opta

Set in 9.5/12pt Meridien by SPi Publisher Services, Pondicherry, India
Printed in Singapore by Ho Printing Singapore Pte Ltd

1   2013

Contents

viii   Contents

Part 4: Lower Urinary Tract

Part 8: Clinical Management

List of contributors

Tev Aho, Consultant Urological Surgeon, Addenbrooke's Hospital, Cambridge, UK

Ben Ayres, SpR Urology, Croydon University Hospital, Croydon, UK

Ruzi Begum, SpR Urology, Heatherwood and Wexham Park Hospital, Slough, UK

Richard Bell, Consultant Urological Surgeon, Northampton General Hospital, Northampton, UK

Jeetesh Bhardwa, SpR Urology, Heatherwood and Wexham Park Hospital, Slough, UK

Anthony Blacker, Consultant Urological Surgeon, University Hospital, Coventry, UK

Simon Bott, Consultant Urological Surgeon, Frimley Park Hospital, Frimley, UK

David Bouchier-Hayes, Consultant Urological Surgeon and Robotic Surgeon, Galway Clinic, Co. Galway, Ireland

Matthew Bultitude, Consultant Urological Surgeon, Guy's and St Thomas' Hospitals, London, UK

Neil Burgess, Consultant Urological Surgeon Norfolk and Norwich University Hospital Norwich, Norfolk, UK

John G. Calleary, Consultant Urological Surgeon, North Manchester General Hospital, Manchester, UK

Jon Cartledge, Consultant Urological Surgeon, St James's University Hospital, Leeds, UK

David Chadwick, Consultant Urological Surgeon, James Cook University Hospital, Middlesbrough, UK

Ben Challacombe, Consultant Urological Surgeon and Honorary Senior Lecturer, Guy's Hospital and King's College London, London, UK

Aasem Chaudry, Consultant Urological Surgeon, Bedford Hospital, Bedford, UK

Justin Collins, Consultant Urological Surgeon, St Peters Hospital, Chertsey, UK

Glyn Constantine, Consultant Gynaecologist, Good Hope Hospital, Sutton Coldfield, UK

Peter W. Cooke, Consultant Urological Surgeon, Royal Wolverhampton Hospitals, Wolverhampton, UK

David Cranston, Consultant Urological Surgeon and Senior Lecturer in Surgery, Churchill Hospital, Oxford, UK

Gary Das, Consultant Urological Surgeon, Croydon University Hospital, Croydon, UK

Prokar Dasgupta, Professor of Robotic Surgery and Urological Innovation, Kings College London, King's Health Partners, London, UK

Andrew Doble, Consultant Urological Surgeon, Addenbrooke's Hospital, Cambridge, UK

Chris Eden, Consultant Urological Surgeon, The Prostate Clinic, The Hampshire Clinic, Basingstoke, UK

Derek Fawcett, Consultant Urological Surgeon, Harold Hopkins Department of Urology, Royal Berkshire NHS Foundation Trust, Reading, UK

Simon Fulford, Consultant Urological Surgeon, James Cook University Hospital, Middlesbrough, UK

Stephen Gordon, Consultant Urological Surgeon, Epsom and St Helier University Hospitals NHS Trust, Surrey, UK

Rob Gray, SpR Urology, Heatherwood and Wexham Park Hospital, Slough, UK

James Hall, Consultant Urological Surgeon, Royal Hallamshire Hospital, Sheffield, UK

Paul Halliday, Consultant Urological Surgeon, Ninewells Hospital, Dundee, UK

Rizwan Hamid, Consultant Urological Surgeon, Royal National Orthopaedic Hospital, Stanmore and University College London Hospitals, London, UK

Damian Hanbury, Consultant Urological Surgeon, Lister Hospital, Stevenage, UK

Neil Harris, Consultant Urological Surgeon, St James' University Hospital, Leeds, UK

Matt Hayes, Consultant Urological Surgeon, Southampton General Hospital, Southhampton, UK

David Hendry, Consultant Urological Surgeon, Gartnavel General Hospital, Glasgow, UK

Dominic Hodgson, Consultant Urological Surgeon, Queen Alexandra Hospital, Portsmouth, UK

Adam Jones, Consultant Urological Surgeon, Harold Hopkins Department of Urology, Royal Berkshire NHS Foundation Trust, Reading, UK

Rob Jones, Consultant Urological Surgeon, Musgrove Park Hospital, Taunton, UK

Omer Karim, Consultant Urological Surgeon, Heatherwood and Wexham Park Hospital, Slough, UK

Patrick F. Keane, Consultant Urological Surgeon, Belfast City Hospital, Belfast, UK

John Kelleher, Consultant Urological Surgeon, Wycombe Hospital, High Wycombe, UK

John D. Kelly, Professor of Urology Honorary Consultant Urological Surgeon University College Hospital, London, UK

Muhammad Jamal Khan, SpR Urology, Heatherwood and Wexham Park Hospital, Slough, UK

Alex Kirkham, Consultant Uroradiologist, University College London Hospitals, London, UK

Pardeep Kumar, Specialist Registrar Urology and Fellow in Uro-Oncology, Royal Marsden Hospital, London, UK

Sunil Kumar, Consultant Urological Surgeon, Harold Hopkins Department of Urology, Royal Berkshire NHS Foundation Trust, Reading and Heatherwood and Wexham Park Hospital, Slough, UK

Marc Laniado, Consultant Urological Surgeon, Heatherwood and Wexham Park Hospital, Slough, UK

Ling Lee, Consultant Urological Surgeon, Royal Bolton Hospital, Bolton, UK

Ru MacDonagh, Consultant Urological Surgeon, Musgrove Park Hospital, Taunton, UK

Peter Malone, Consultant Urological Surgeon, Harold Hopkins Department of Urology, Royal Berkshire NHS Foundation Trust, Reading, UK

Paul McInerney, Consultant Urological Surgeon, Derriford Hospital, Plymouth, UK

John McLoughlin, Consultant Urological Surgeon, West Suffolk Hospital, Bury St Edmunds, UK

Alan McNeill, Consultant Urological Surgeon, Western General Hospital, Edinburgh, UK

Suks Minhas, Consultant Uro-Andrologist, University College London Hospitals, London, UK

Hanif Motiwala, Consultant Urological Surgeon, Heatherwood and Wexham Park Hospital, Slough, UK

K Mozolowski, CT1 Urology Trainee, NW Deanery, North Manchester General Hospital, Manchester, UK

Asif Muneer, Consultant Urological Surgeon and Andrologist, University College London Hospitals, London, UK

Richard Napier-Hemy, Consultant Urological Surgeon, Manchester Royal Infirmary, Manchester, UK

Senthil Nathan, Consultant Urological Surgeon, Whittington Hospital, London and Institute of Urology, University College London Hospitals, London, UK

J. Curtis Nickel, Consultant Urological Surgeon, Queen's University, Kingston, ON, Canada

David Nicol, Consultant Urological Surgeon, Royal Free Hospital, London, UK

Edgar Paez, SpR Urology, Freeman Hospital, Newcastle upon Tyne, UK

Toby Page, Consultant Urological Surgeon, Freeman Hospital, Newcastle upon Tyne, UK

Bo Parys, Consultant Urological Surgeon, Rotherham District General Hospital, Rotherham, UK

Jhumur Pati, Consultant Urological Surgeon, Barts and the London Hospital, London, UK

Amjad Mumtaz Peracha, Consultant Urological Surgeon, Royal Derby Hospitals, Derby, UK

Asif Raza, Consultant Urological Surgeon, Ealing Hospital, Middlesex and Charing Cross Hospitals, London, UK

Tony Riddick, Consultant Urological Surgeon, Western General Hospital, Edinburgh, UK

Peter Rimmington, Consultant Urological Surgeon, Eastbourne District General Hospital, Eastbourne, UK

Gerald Rix, Consultant Urological Surgeon, Colchester Hospital, Colchester, UK

Simon Robinson, SpR Urology, Heatherwood and Wexham Park Hospital, Slough, UK

Henry Sells, Consultant Urological Surgeon, Derriford Hospital, Plymouth, UK

Nimish Shah, Consultant Urological Surgeon, Addenbrooke's Hospital, Cambridge, UK

Rajindra Singh, SpR Urology, Barts and the London Hospital, London, UK

Graham Sole, Consultant Urological Surgeon, Hereford County Hospital, Hereford, UK

Mark J. Speakman, Consultant Urological Surgeon, Musgrove Park Hospital, Taunton, UK

Stephanie J. Symons, Consultant Urological Surgeon, Pinderfields Hospital, Mid Yorkshire NHS Trust, Wakefield, UK

Nikesh Thiruchelvam, Consultant Urological Surgeon, Addenbrooke's Hospital, Cambridge, UK

Andrew C. Thorpe, Consultant Urological Surgeon, Freeman Hospital, Newcastle upon Tyne, UK

Philip van Kerrebroeck, Professor of Urology, University of Maastricht, Maastricht, The Netherlands

Nikhil Vasdev, Consultant Urological Surgeon, James Cook University Hospital, Middlesbrough, UK

Dan Wilby, SpR Urology, Southampton General Hospital, Southampton, UK

Georgina Wilson, Consultant Urological Surgeon, West Suffolk Hospital, Bury St Edmunds, UK

Oliver Wiseman, Consultant Urological Surgeon, Addenbrooke's Hospital, Cambridge, UK

Dan Wood, Consultant Adolescent and Reconstructive Urological Surgeon, University College London Hospitals, London, UK

Sarah Wood, Consultant Urological Surgeon, Norfolk and Norwich University Hospital, Norwich, UK

Christopher Woodhouse, Emeritus Professor of Adolescent Urology, University College London and Consultant Urologist, Royal Marsden Hospital, London, UK

Lehana Yeo, ST4 Urology, Barts and the London Hospital, London, UK

Foreword

'You can't teach an old dog new tricks' and I am about as old a dog as you can get! Actually, I have learnt a few new tricks and, what is more, my cynical expectation that they would all, actually, be old tricks that have been rediscovered, has proved to be unfounded.

When John McLoughlin produced the first edition of this book I thought it was an interesting idea, and a second edition is entirely justified by the huge expansion in laparoscopic and robotic urology since that first edition. There are tips and tricks here that are no more than one sentence long and so this is an easy book to pick up and browse as well as to search for an answer to a particular point.

It is interesting to see the number of tips that include the comment 'I learnt this tip from …'. I suspect that in the book as a whole we therefore have the collective memory of British Urology.

I thought this was not just an interesting book but an intellectually amusing one as well, and for that reason I heartily recommend it to urologists anywhere and everywhere.

Anthony R. Mundy
PhD(Hon) MS FRCP FRCS
Professor of Urology
Institute of Urology, London, UK

Preface

This is not a textbook. It is intended to pass on useful tips, operative manoeuvres or pearls of wisdom from experienced urologists that may not otherwise find their way into standard urological texts. At its heart are those questions which trainees ask their senior colleagues, such as 'What would you do when…?' or 'How do you like to do it?'. By their nature the replies are quirky, and often personal.

Wherever possible, the text has not been altered from the original, other than removal of references and diagrams professionally redrawn.

Sadly, we felt unable to accept the anonymous contribution that read 'My top tip is to always place the wheel barrow in the direction of travel before filling it with soil'. At the end are included a few quotes that were sent in. They don't really fit into any particular category but are worth reading.

John McLoughlin
Neil Burgess
Hanif Motiwala
Mark J. Speakman
Andrew Doble
John Kelly

List of abbreviations

AP	anteroposterior; abdomino-perineal resection
ASIS	anterior superior iliac spine
BMI	Body Mass Index
BNI	bladder neck incision
BXO	balanitis xerotica obliterans
CP	chronic prostatitis
CPPS	chronic pelvic pain syndrome
CT	computed tomography
DRE	digital rectal examination
DVC	dorsal vein complex
EAU	European Association of Urology
FC	flexible cystoscope
GA	general anaesthetic
IPSS	International Prostate Symptom Score
IVC	inferior vena cava
LUTS	lower urinary tract symptoms
MRI	magnetic resonance imaging
MSU	midstream urine
NIH-CPSI	NIH Chronic Prostatitis Symptom Index
OP	open prostatectomy
PCCL	percutaneous cystolithotomy
PCNL	percutaneous nephrolithotomy
PS	pubic symphysis
PSA	prostate-specific antigen
PUJ	pelvi-ureteric junction
RALP	robotic-assisted laparoscopic pyeloplasty
RARC	robotic-assisted radical cystectomy
RARP	robotic-assisted radical prostatectomy
RP	radical prostatectomy
SUI	stress urinary incontinence
TCC	transitional cell carcinoma
TURBT	transurethral resection of bladder tumour
TURP	transurethral resection of prostate
TWOC	trial without catheter
UO	ureteric orifices
US	urethral stump
VUJ	vesico-ureteric junction

PART 1
Open Urology

Top Tips in Urology, Second Edition. Edited by John McLoughlin, Neil Burgess, Hanif Motiwala, Mark J. Speakman, Andrew Doble and John D. Kelly.
© 2013 John Wiley & Sons, Ltd. Published 2013 by John Wiley & Sons, Ltd.

1

A technique to minimise the risk of ureteric injury in patients with an enlarged median lobe undergoing radical prostatectomy

Nikhil Vasdev and David Chadwick

With an increasing number of patients undergoing radical prostatic surgery (laparoscopic, robotic and open) for prostate cancer worldwide, there continues to be an increasing risk of ureteric injury. The risk is minimised with adequate identification of the ureteric orifices.

We present a 'top tip' of performing a cystoscopy and cannulating both ureteric orifices (UO) prior to performing prostatic surgery in patients with an enlarged median lobe in order to minimise the risk of inadvertent injury to the UO while opening the bladder during a radical prostatectomy (RP). The technique involves a cystoscopy and cannulation of both UO with ureteric catheters (Figure 1.1). The patient is then operated on using the planned technique of radical prostatectomy (laparoscopic, robotic and open) and the ureteric catheters are identified on opening of the bladder neck. Upon

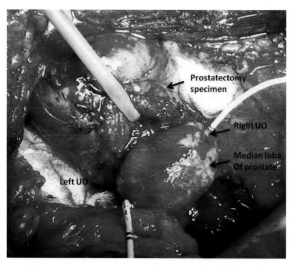

Figure 1.1 Open radical prostatectomy with large median lobe and laterally situated ureteric orifices.

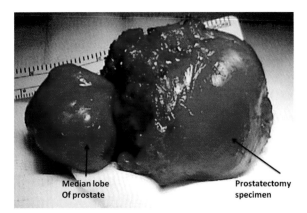

Figure 1.2 Radical prostatectomy specimen with enlarged median lobe.

completion of this step the bladder neck and UOs are clearly identified at the time of excision of the prostate specimen and bladder reconstruction. We advocate this step to prevent inadvertent ureteric injury. Using this technique, the incidence of ureteric injury at our centre in patients undergoing open RP is 0.06% (1/1500). A demonstration of the median lobe is presented in Figure 1.2.

2

Novel methods to aid vesicourethral anastomosis in radical retropubic prostatectomy

Lehana Yeo, Rajindra Singh and Jhumur Pati

Vesicourethral anastomosis is a technically challenging aspect of retropubic radical prostatectomy. Here are two novel and inexpensive methods that may be used to facilitate anastomosis of the urethral stump to the bladder neck where direct visualisation of the stump is difficult (e.g. prominent bony spur or retracted urethral stump).

The first involves use of an anterior dental mirror. The mirror is typically angulated, providing indirect vision of the catheterised stump (Figure 2.1). Pretreatment of the mirror with an anti-fog prevents condensation.

The second involves insertion of a flexible cystoscope per urethra with irrigation running. Under direct vision, the cystoscope is advanced to the level of the transected urethra. Illumination from the cystoscope improves the view, produces telescoping of the retracted urethra and also angulation of the urethral stump, thus providing a clear view of the transected urethra.

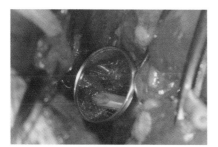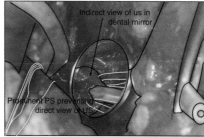

Figure 2.1 Use of dental mirror to achieve indirect vision of the urethral stump (US). Pubic symphysis (PS). (Reproduced with permission from Lehana Y, Rajindra S, Jhumur P: Novel Methods to Aid Vesicourethral Anastomosis in Radical Retropubic Prostatectomy. Curr Urol 2011;5:209–212, S. Karger AG Basel.)

Our preference for construction of the anastomosis involves placing six sutures into the urethal stump at 2, 4, 6, 8, 10 and 12 o'clock positions. No special equipment is required as most theatres possess a dental mirror and both tips avoid the need for the patient to be put into the lithotomy position in order to allow direct perineal pressure.

The use of the flexible cystoscope would also be beneficial in laparoscopic or robotic prostatectomy.

3

Surgical technique to reduce intraoperative bleeding during open prostatectomy

Nikhil Vasdev, Edgar Paez and Andrew C. Thorpe

Open prostatectomy (OP) is indicated in patients with large benign adenomas of the prostate which are not amenable to current transurethral resection techniques. Despite its proven efficiency, OP is associated with a risk of intra- and perioperative bleeding, related to the rich arterial and venous supply of the prostate gland.

We recommend the use of the HARMONIC wave scalpel (Figure 3.1) during OP to reduce the risk of bleeding. Our technique recommends two steps. The initial step is the application of a row of interrupted Vicryl 2/0 sutures on the prostatic capsule and the second step involves the application of the HARMONIC wave scalpel to open the prostatic capsule (Figure 3.2).

We used this technique in 30 patients between May 2007 and July 2011. In our series, the mean size of prostate adenoma at the time of surgery was 118 cm³ (range 83–400). The computed tomography scan of a large benign prostatic adenoma with a volume of 400 cm³ is demonstrated in Figure 3.3. Sixteen percent (5/30) of patients required a blood transfusion (intraopera-

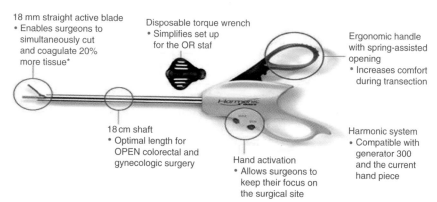

Figure 3.1 HARMONIC wave scalpel. (Courtesy of Ms Helen Leith, Energy Specialist, Ethicon Endo-Surgery, Johnson & Johnson, UK.)

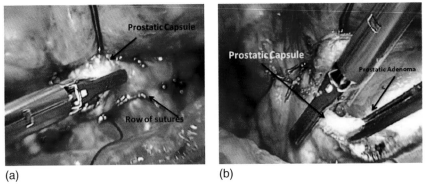

(a)   (b)

Figure 3.2 (a) Initial application of sutures. (b) Opening of prostatic capsule.

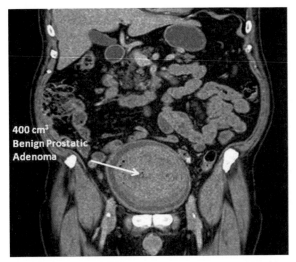

Figure 3.3 Large benign prostatic adenoma from our series, measuring 400 cm³.

tive and postoperative). The rate of blood transfusion before the introduction of this technique was 45% (9/20) in our previous series.

Our technique reduces the incidence of intra-/postoperative blood transfusion and enhances an early discharge after OP.

4

Millin's prostatectomy

Rob Jones and Ru MacDonagh

Open retropubic prostatectomy has become a dying art, sadly; we feel this procedure still has a role when the prostate is very large indeed and can be both more effective and safer than transurethral surgery. The following three tips were passed on by Professor Paul Abrams, who had himself inherited them from Roger Feneley, and have proved themselves invaluable in our experience.

1 Having fully exposed the prostate capsule, put a 0 Vicryl stay suture at each end of the planned capsulotomy (a figure-of-eight suture placed as laterally as possible, tie and leave the needle on). These sutures mark the limit of the subsequent capsular incision; most importantly, they prevent further tearing of the capsule during adenoma enucleation and also allow for easy closure afterwards.

2 Having incised the prostate capsule down to the 'adenoma', the midline anterior commissure can easily be identified by passing an 18F Clutton sound transurethrally, then bluntly pushing it through into the capsulotomy anteriorly. This allows the index finger to enter the prostatic lumen for adenoma enucleation.

3 In order to protect the urethral sphincter, the adenoma is most safely enucleated in a retrograde manner. Feel first for the verumontanum and the prostatic apex before peeling the prostate back towards the bladder neck. This releases the sphincter at an early stage and prevents it from damage by being inadvertently pulled up with the prostate, thereby limiting the risk of sphincter weakness incontinence.

5

Cystectomy

Patrick F. Keane

During cystectomy, several important planes are developed. Once vascular pedicles have been identified and the posterior plane is fully developed, the vascular pedicles and connective tissue attachments to the rectum can be divided in seconds with the stapling device (Figures 5.1 and 5.2). In the 'difficult pelvis' and obese patients, it is particularly useful and the end of the device is articulated for ease of firing. If the pedicle to be divided is very thick then a pause before firing allows any oedema in the tissue to be stapled to dissipate.

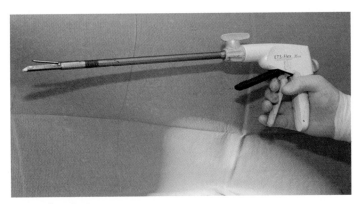

Figure 5.1 Stapling device.

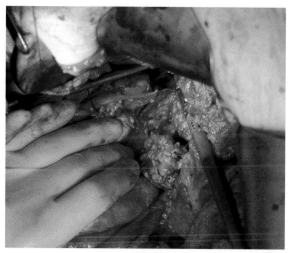

Figure 5.2 View into pelvis with device deployed.

6

Salvage cystectomy and prostatectomy

Senthil Nathan

In salvage operations of the prostate and bladder following radiotherapy, there may be dense adhesions between the bladder and prostate and the rectum. Frequently, tiny perforations in the rectum can occur. These may go unrecognised during surgery and to avoid this, the rectum should be filled with methylene blue before the operation.

7

Creating an ileal conduit spout

Simon Fulford

Creating a good spout on an ileal conduit is vital for ease of future management and will impress your stoma nurse! It can, however, be difficult, particularly in an obese patient. I have found the following techniques helpful.

1 Where possible, divide the mesentery in such a way that rather than being perpendicular to the distal end of the conduit, it is angled at about 45° to the bowel – this reduces the bulk of mesentery that is pulled through the abdominal wall.

2 Make a cruciate incision in the rectus fascia and place a Vicryl suture into each of the four triangular flaps produced before splitting the muscle and peritoneum and pulling the conduit through.

3 Gently pull as much conduit through as you can whilst feeding it out of the abdomen with your other hand. If it feels too short, try bringing it through the gap in the ileal mesentery created when you isolated the conduit – this sometimes gives you an extra couple of centimetres.

4 With the conduit pulled through as much as possible, take your four prepositioned sutures and use them to anchor the serosa to the rectus fascial flaps.

5 Take four more sutures at the four points of the compass (N, S, E, W) and pass through skin edge, serosa 2–3 cm from the end of the conduit and serosa at the end of the conduit. Place each in a clip and then pull all four simultaneously. You should now get a spout. Tie the four sutures then add sutures in between to complete the stoma.

6 If ileum is not going to reach the surface comfortably whatever you do or is badly affected by radiotherapy or disease, use large bowel. The marginal artery allows a mesentery free stoma to be created and the transverse colon is unlikely to be affected by pelvic radiotherapy.

8

Prefashioning a urostomy

Richard Bell

Prefashion the urostomy prior to pulling it through the abdominal wall. This technique was originally shown to me by Paul McInerney (Plymouth) some years ago, and reliably produces a healthy protruding urostomy spout.

See Figures 8.1–8.3.

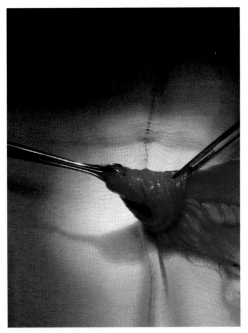

Figure 8.1 Gently evert using a Babcock forceps.

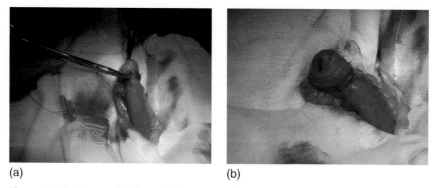

(a)   (b)

Figure 8.2 (a) Secure in place with interrupted sutures. (b) Prepared conduit prior to pulling through abdominal wall. A nice spout has been easily achieved.

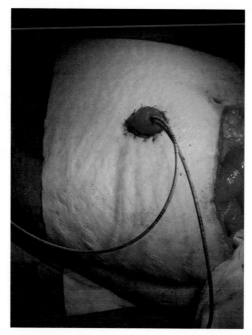

Figure 8.3 Appearance of the final conduit (with ureteric catheters in place).

9

A novel technique for parastomal hernia repair

Jeetesh Bhardwa, Rob Gray and Hanif Motiwala

Parastomal hernias are a problematic issue. Recurrent ones are really trouble-some. Here is a technique which we have found very useful for parastomal hernias, including those from ileal conduit urinary diversion or from colostomy.

An incision is marked around the stoma and extended on both sides (Figure 9.1a, b). This is dipping down to the level of the rectus sheath and hernia needs to be reduced after proper dissection. The rectus sheath is incised all around the hernia and secured as a first layer of securing the hernia around the stoma. Parietene Progrip mesh (a self-sticking mesh) is secured and placed as a corset on top of it (like a Polo mint) and is then secured to the rectus sheath as well as the stoma wall (Figure 9.2).

In our opinion, this provides double strength and prevents future recurrences, firstly by securing the rectus sheath and also by using the Parietene Progrip mesh. Our personal experience of this technique has been very successful for both primary and recurrent parastomal hernia cases.

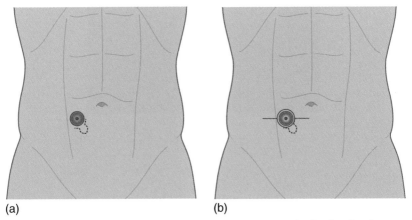

(a)   (b)

Figure 9.1 (a) Stoma with parastomal hernia. (b) Incision. (Abridged and redrawn from Ho KM, Fawcett DP. Parastomal hernia repair using the lateral approach. British Journal of Urology International 2004; 94: 598–602.)

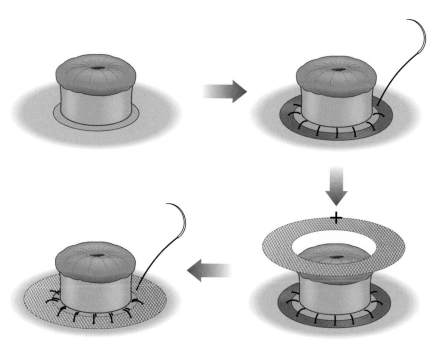

Figure 9.2 Incision of rectus sheath, folding of rectus sheath parastomally and reinforcement using Parietene Progrip mesh. (Abridged and redrawn from Ho KM, Fawcett DP. Parastomal hernia repair using the lateral approach. British Journal of Urology International 2004; 94: 598–602.)

10

Parastomal hernia repair

Derek Fawcett

A parastomal hernia after ileal conduit formation is probably more frequent than many urologists acknowledge. The hernia tends to occur at the superolateral quadrant (9–12 o'clock position) of the stoma site in the right iliac fossa. The mesentery normally lies at the 2–3 o'clock position of the stoma, the superolateral quadrant representing an area of little resistance where the abdominal content can easily herniate. The indications for surgery include pain, cosmesis and risk of bowel obstruction or strangulation.

The lateral approach described here obviates the need for laparotomy and stomal relocation, and allows continued use of the usual stoma appliance as there is no peristomal incision. The dissection stays medial onto the external oblique fascia. Extra care is needed in managing the very large and difficult hernia so as to avoid devascularising the conduit.

The procedure should be covered with intravenous antibiotics, continued for three doses after surgery. The patient should be placed in the supine position and urine temporarily diverted from the wound by inserting a Foley catheter into the conduit. The stoma in turn should be protected from the wound by a gauze swab and drape.

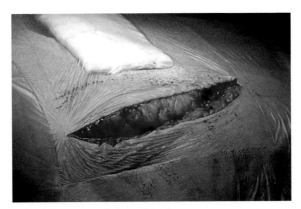

Figure 10.1 The incision was made lateral to the stoma.

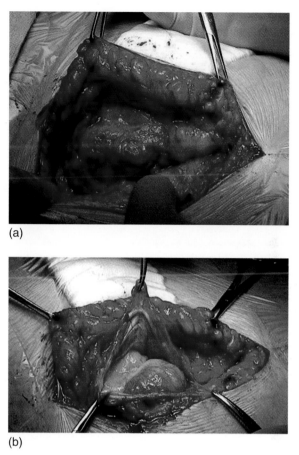

(a)

(b)

Figure 10.2 (a,b) Identification and opening of the hernia sac.

A lateral incision is made about 10 cm from the stoma through the skin into the subcutaneous tissue, well lateral to the stomahesive skin marks (Figure 10.1). The extent of the hernia defect is delineated and the hernia sac carefully preserved (Figure 10.2a). After extraperitoneal reduction of the hernia content, the defect is closed with interrupted non-absorbable sutures. Alternatively, the sac can be opened (Figure 10.2b) and the content reduced into the peritoneal cavity before the defect is closed with interrupted sutures. The closed defect is then reinforced with a prosthetic mesh (Prolene, Ethicon, UK), tailored to cover the lateral aspect (6–12 o'clock position) of the stoma (Figure 10.3). The mesh is secured by interrupted non-absorbable sutures onto the external oblique fascia. A drain is left around the mesh before wound closure (Figure 10.4).

Without using a mesh repair the hernia recurrence rate is much higher. As the lateral approach obviates the need for laparotomy and stomal relocation,

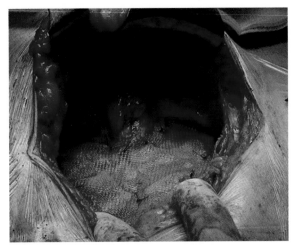

Figure 10.3 The mesh used for reinforcing the hernia. The conduit lies medial to the mesh.

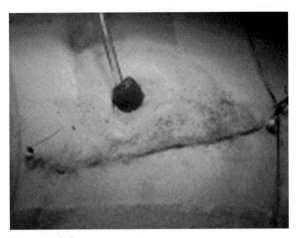

Figure 10.4 After wound closure.

it enhances a quick return of bowel function, early discharge and early recovery.

The anatomical landmarks and surgical principles described here can also be of value when contemplating laparoscopic hernia parastomal repair.

11

Nephrectomy: vascular control during caval thrombectomy

Dan Wilby and Matt Hayes

Traditionally, techniques to control major vessels during retroperitoneal surgery have involved the use of metal vascular clamps. Although engineered to be atraumatic, these clamps can potentially injure the walls of fragile veins, often in areas that are difficult to access. The use of vascular slings combined with tubes (snuggers) and mosquito clips minimises trauma to the vessel wall whilst providing effective vascular control; their flexibility also minimises intrusion into the operative field.

Once the vessel wall is circumferentially accessible, e.g. using Lahey forceps, the vessel can be slung, both free ends of the sling passed through the snugger, the snugger applied firmly to the wall of the vessel and secured using a mosquito forceps (Figure 11.1). Care should be taken to incorporate the vessel only and to ensure that arterial /venous ischaemia is minimised according to organ sensitivity to ischaemia.

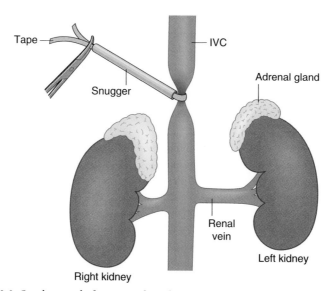

Figure 11.1 Good control of cava can be achieved by snugger and mosquito clamp.

12

Secure ligation of foreshortened large veins

Dan Wilby and Matt Hayes

It can be difficult to ligate and divide short vessels leaving an adequate cuff to prevent the ligature slipping off. Often the ligature will slip on the vessel as it is tightened, resulting in inaccurate placement of the tie. In order to better control the placement of ties in such a situation, we recommend a second pass of the ligature around the vessel that secures it in the desired location before it is tied. An added benefit of this technique is a more even circumferential distribution of forces within the ligature, ensuring secure ligation of the vessel and reducing the risk of cheese-wiring.

13

How to avoid dislodging the vascular clamp

Asif Muneer

When applying a Satinsky clamp to major vessels, there is always the danger of the clamp inadvertently becoming loose and dislodging, resulting in catastrophic haemorrhage.

Once the clamp has been applied, tie a 0 Vicryl suture through the handles and this will secure the clamp. Once vascular control has been achieved, the suture can be cut and the clamp released.

14

Ligating the renal artery

David Cranston

My best tip for ligating the renal artery in complex renal surgery is to get a finger and thumb around the whole renal hilum and then follow that with a Satinsky clamp which I make sure touches my finger as I guide it around (to avoid making a hole in anything I should not). I put a 1.0 Vicryl into the Satinsky and bring it back so that the suture is around the hilum (artery and vein). I then carefully mobilise the vein and, again with finger and thumb, get under the vein alone, and take the appropriate end of the Vicryl under the vein and tie it. This means that the artery is ligated – but not the vein at this stage – without the need to dissect or identify the artery separately. You can feel the pulsation so you know where it is.

15

Renal hypothermia using an innovative ice sludge technique

Ruzi Begum and Hanif Motiwala

Open renal surgery using renal hypothermia is very well known and despite the emergence of new technology using robotics and laparoscopy, it has a role to play in larger renal tumours, renal tumours at mid pole requiring reconstruction or large staghorn stones requiring anatrophic nephrolithotomy and reconstruction.

There are commercially available bags for use in this situation but over the last few years we have used a urine bag for this purpose and the photographs here show where we cut and divide the bag (Figures 15.1 and 15.2). It is cheap and readily available. It also provides good temperature control to avoid body hypothermia.

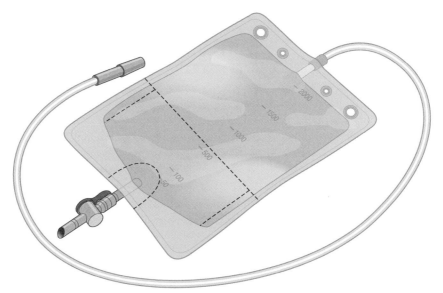

Figure 15.1 Standard urine catheter bag.

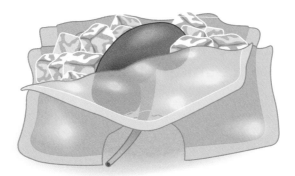

Figure 15.2 Opened catheter bag with ice surrounding the kidney.

16

Making the best of a short suture length in a deep dark hole

John McLoughlin

When working down in a deep hole, you will occasionally complete a suture line with only a short length remaining, which you need to use to throw your knot. While you can struggle to tie the knot with what is usually a short loop

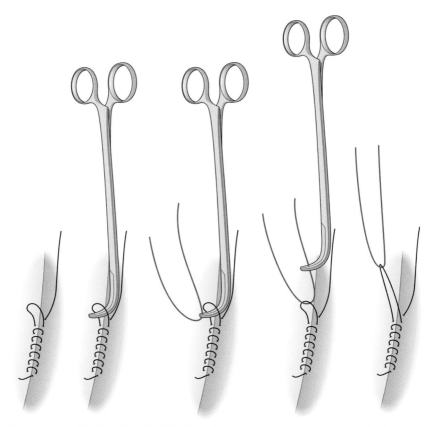

Figure 16.1 Pull a short length of tie through a loop in a short suture using, for instance, a Roberts forceps. Once the knot has been tied, the extra length can be removed.

of suture, a simpler solution is to slip a length of any available suture (e.g. Vicryl) through the loop using a pair of right-angled forceps. This in effect provides an extension of your suture, allowing you to throw the knot, and it can then be pulled out before cutting the end of the length (Figure 16.1). It only takes a few seconds but will save a lot of aggravation.

17

Anterior approach for a pyeloplasty

John McLoughlin

Some years ago I undertook a pyeloplasty on a woman with a horseshoe kidney. I found references to an anterior extraperitoneal approach. I loved it and have used it ever since for slim, small-build, little old ladies (not fat or muscular men!). Selection is the key!

Perform a retrograde study in the lithotomy position with the C-arm over top. Fill up the renal pelvis with contrast and mark the level of the pelvi-ureteric junction (PUJ) on the anterior abdominal wall with a marker pen using a long line from lateral to medial (Figure 17.1, line X-X). Then, rotate the C-arm through 90° and place a metal clip on your mark to really make sure it is at the precise level of the PUJ. This is important. Then, put the legs down and recheck that the PUJ hasn't moved from the mark point. Put a sandbag under the kidney and recheck one last time. If you are happy that the PUJ is located precisely, place the patient in a supine position and draw out the lateral edge of the rectus with the marker pen (see Figure 17.1, line Y-Y).

Make a small muscle-splitting transverse incision lateral to the outer margin of the rectus. Typically 2 inches is enough (see Figure 17.1, line Z-Z). You can use a Langenbeck retractor or a really narrow Deaver; often finding a small enough, deep retractor is a source of frustration. Stay extra-peritoneal and lateral. Take your time and push the peritoneum anteriorly and use a pledget to dissect out tissue planes until you see the ureter. Don't open anything that looks like the peritoneum. If you enter the peritoneum this procedure becomes very tedious. Sling the ureter and use traction to pull it up. Use a pledget to push off the fascial layers surrounding the renal pelvis. As you do, you will see the PUJ and pelvis emerge in a way you never see through the loin! It will, with patience, come right up into the wound, often to near skin level. Place stay sutures around the renal pelvis as it will otherwise retract into oblivion once you open it. Once you have performed your pyeloplasty (plus stent), it is easy to close with interrupted Vicryl.

Typically these patients go home after 24h but I have had one or two go home the next morning. Only rarely do they require anything other than oral

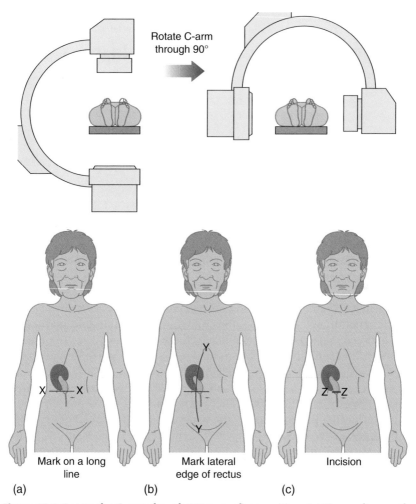

Figure 17.1 Rotate the C-arm though 90° to confirm position. (a) Draw a line on the skin from flank to midline. (b) Draw a line to mark the lateral border of the rectus. (c) The actual incision.

analgesia after the first day. Even in a world of laparoscopic pyeloplasty, I remain impressed with how little systemic interference this causes in these little old ladies.

18

Ureteric injuries – lower third: adaptations of the Boari flap

John Kelleher

We are all familiar with the call from fellow abdominal surgeons, usually gynaecologists: 'I think I have damaged a ureter, can you help me?'. This may be noticed during the primary procedure or later. This tip can apply to either but will be described as if the patient is in the postoperative period of the primary procedure.

Lower third injuries, particularly those identified late, are not clean-cut lacerations. Most commonly, we are faced with a ureter that has been ligated, crushed or sutured into a neighbouring structure. The patient usually has a urine leak into a drain, through the vault of the transected vagina following hysterectomy, or more rarely through the vaginal os following caesarean section.

When faced with this situation, a computed tomography (CT) urogram is invaluable, identifying the level of the injury. The patient is taken to theatre and, with the legs up, has a preliminary cystoscopy and retrograde ureterogram to confirm the diagnosis of ureteric trauma, and importantly to rule out bladder damage. Once the side and level of the injury are known, the legs can be put flat and the patient prepared for exploration. It is helpful to place a sandbag underneath the pelvis on the affected side.

If a Pfannensteil incision has been previously employed, then it is best to extend this in a 'J' shaped fashion up the edge of the rectus abdominis for about 5–10 cm in a cephalad direction. The beauty of this incision is that it is an atraumatic and bloodless entry into the retroperitoneum. After reflecting the peritoneum and its contents medially, one quickly comes across the ureter as it enters the pelvis. It is usually dilated and can be followed easily to the level of the injury. Most ureteric injuries are at the level of the superior vesical artery, and this may need to be divided to gain better access. Also, the round ligament is best divided at this stage in order to gain best access to the bladder.

If the ureter is badly damaged or the level of injury is higher than expected, direct reimplantation into the bladder is not possible because of lack of ureteric length, and this is where the Boari flap comes into its own. In preparing the flap, I fill the bladder from below, running in about 500 mL of saline. The flap is best mapped out after pushing the perivesical fat away and exposing the detrusor muscle. The flap is then fashioned after drawing its outline on the detrusor muscle with the finger touch diathermy, making sure that the base is broad relative to the tip and that there is ample length to reach the distal ureter without any tension.

If necessary, the contralateral superior vesicle pedicle can be divided to gain additional bladder mobility to increase the length of the flap. If the bladder is big I have been able to bring the flap over the pelvic brim to repair a middle third ureteric injury without difficulty.

The flap is then raised and the bladder emptied. The ureter is brought through the distal flap and sutured into position. A ureteric stent is then positioned from kidney to bladder. The bladder is then closed in two layers with absorbable sutures. The wound can be closed. Make sure that you connect the catheter to a drainage bag before the patient is moved to recovery!

This is an incredibly reliable reconstruction. I have never had a urine leak following this procedure and the patients can be discharged safely within 2–3 days and return for a trial without catheter (TWOC) 10 days after surgery. The stent can be removed under local with the flexible cystoscope at 4–6 weeks.

See Figures 18.1–18.5.

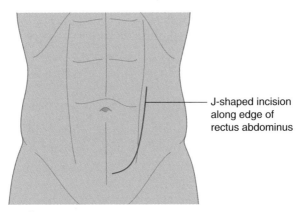

J-shaped incision
along edge of
rectus abdominus

Figure 18.1 Site of incision.

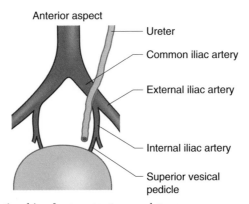

Anterior aspect

Ureter

Common iliac artery

External iliac artery

Internal iliac artery

Superior vesical
pedicle

Figure 18.2 Relationship of cut ureter to vasculature.

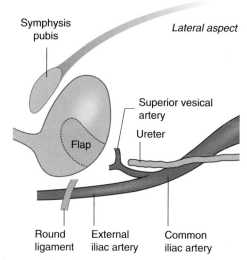

Figure 18.3 Sagittal section from the side.

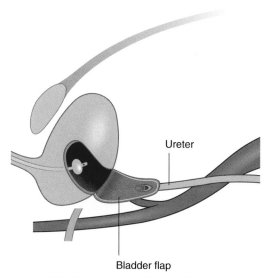

Figure 18.4 The catheterised bladder has been fashioned into a tube to reach the ureter.

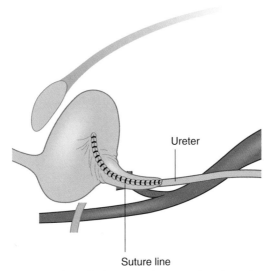

Ureter

Suture line

Figure 18.5 The finished article with the suture line running along the bladder wall into the lower end of the ureter.

19

Radical orchidectomy for germ cell tumours

David Hendry

I heard from Tim Christmas that when a radical orchidectomy for a germ cell tumour is being performed, a non-absorbable transfixion suture should be used at the deep inguinal ring; this means that if the patient goes on to require a retroperitoneal node dissection for metastatic disease, you can be certain of complete excision of all the testicular vessels, because you can see the non-absorbable suture at the end of the dissected specimen. I have been trying to hammer this into all the trainees in the west of Scotland, and as some of them move on to consultant jobs, there are a few patients who come up for their retroperitoneal dissection who have had a non-absorbable suture and it does make life easier.

20

Don't lose the lumen at urethroplasty

Andrew Doble

Prior to urethroplasty, urethroscopy and placement of a Sensor guidewire into the bladder will prevent loss of the lumen when the stricture is opened. The technique is employed for optical urethrotomy so why not for open surgery? After placement, the guidewire is fixed with a suture to the prepuce or penile shaft.

21

Emergency call to the gynae/obstetric theatre

John McLoughlin

Over the years I have on occasion been called to the gynae/obstetric theatre. Here are a few tips I have learned.

1 Usually the patient is catheterised. Ask. If she is not, then do so as you may otherwise struggle to get a view.

2 Take time to stop the bleeding before you begin. This sounds obvious but unless you do, you will just sit in a sea of ooze and struggle. Don't use suction – at least initially. Instead, put a series of large packs in and apply a little pressure whilst getting organised.

3 Request your usual instruments. Take out the gynae retractors and put in something you are happy with. Theirs are often less than useful. I like the self-retaining Book-Walter. I use a head light. I like to use a 5/8th Monocryl suture which has a lovely circumference that allows the tip to present itself back to you once it has passed through the tissue and it is great for under-running large veins.

4 Take the packs out, one at a time, and make sure each bleeding point is secured before you remove the next. I have seen bleeding from a number of unexpected non-urological places including the vaginal vault, uterine pedicles and iliacs.

5 Get the surgeon to talk you through their anatomy to orientate you. Once they have done so, have a look yourself and make your own mind up.

6 If it is the ureter that is possibly damaged, start upstream and away from the area in question and identify it somewhere safe to sling it. Only then trace it down to the area where injury is suspected. Use the sling to gently put countertraction on the ureter to help identify anatomy. Check both sides!

7 Usually you will be looking into a Pfannensteil incision. If you cannot get a good enough view despite adequate retraction then ask yourself 'Am I happy with the incision?'. You can extend it upwards along the lateral border of the rectus. This is especially important if you are exploring a ureteric injury several days after the event as the ureter may have retracted up out of the pelvis if it has been transected, in a manner similar to cutting an elastic band.

8 I have seen the bladder opened inadvertently and stitched into the uterus as the uterus is closed at emergency caesarean section. Don't be tempted to open the uterus to retrieve it. The problem usually arose because of panic due to excess bleeding. You will regret opening the uterus! Simply excise it and leave as little on view as possible, then close the bladder as usual.

9 If there is a need to distend the bladder, for example prior to formation of a Boari flap, I like to use a 1 L bag of saline with 500 mL of the contents run out prior to connecting it to the catheter. If you keep the tap open, you can both elevate and fill the bladder, or alternatively lower the bag onto the floor and empty it intermittently if you need to empty the bladder or use it as a catheter drainage bag temporarily. This also flushes out the clots from the bladder into the wound before you close a perforation. Unless the bag is half empty at the beginning, you can't do this.

10 You may need to extend the antibiotic cover beyond what is already on board (e.g. vaginal and bladder injury during caesarean section).

11 Instillation of methylene blue into the bladder via the catheter helps if you need to check bladder wall integrity beyond simply running in saline.

12 Make sure that the postoperative plans are clearly written by you. The gynae team may need written advice about when to remove a catheter or stent or details of when to arrange a cystogram.

13 Last but not least, don't be embarrassed – ask all the 'onlookers' who will have accumulated in theatre to leave so as to reduce the noise and clutter.

22

Is it urine in the drain?

Christopher Woodhouse

When relatively clear fluid is flowing from a surgical drain or from the vagina, there is often a concern that it may be urine. Usually, a sample is sent to the lab with a request for creatinine measurement. It may then be 'lost' or the lab may be unsure how it should be labelled in the results file.

It is simpler and much quicker to do a 'Dextrostix' on it and then, if necessary, compare it to a Dextrostix on the blood. If they are the same, it is serum. If there is no glucose in the drainage fluid, it is urine.

23

Cutaneous fistula

Senthil Nathan

Frequently, this is a clinical dilemma in a ward round. The fluid coming out of the abdomen is either urine or serous fluid or there is a faecal fistula. The worrying problem is always faecal fistula and if the fluid is tested for bile acids with a dipstick then it will confirm this to be of enteric content. Biochemical analysis will differentiate between urine and serum.

24

Postoperative abdominal drain

Senthil Nathan

Following operations on the bladder, cystectomy and radical prostatectomy, an abdominal drain is left *in situ*. The internal diameter of this drain is much larger than the urinary catheter. Thus, if the drain is left to hang on the side of the bed below the patient's body, it will create a suction effect (similar to a toilet flush) and suck all the urine towards it, diverting it away from the urinary catheter. This will cause the urinary leak to persist. The drain should be left on top of the bed and the urinary catheter on the side of the bed.

PART 2

Laparoscopic and Robotic Urology

Top Tips in Urology, Second Edition. Edited by John McLoughlin, Neil Burgess,
Hanif Motiwala, Mark J. Speakman, Andrew Doble and John D. Kelly.
© 2013 John Wiley & Sons, Ltd. Published 2013 by John Wiley & Sons, Ltd.

25

Modified Hassan technique in super-obese patients

Tev Aho

The standard Hassan technique may not be possible in super-obese patients due to length limitations of the standard retractors and instruments. If a visual port is not available the following technique can be used to obtain safe initial peritoneal access using the Hassan principles.

- Plan to use the initial port site as the final extraction site and extend the skin incision as much as necessary in the appropriate direction.
- Use appropriately wide and deep retractors (e.g. large Langenbeck, Kelly) to retract each layer in turn as the incisions in fascia and muscle are opened and spread down to preperitoneal fat.

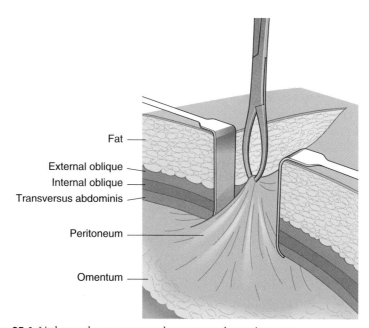

Figure 25.1 Littlewoods retractor used to tent up the peritoneum.

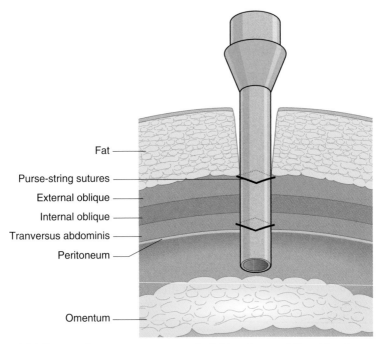

Fat

Purse-string sutures

External oblique

Internal oblique

Tranversus abdominis

Peritoneum

Omentum

Figure 25.2 Purse-string sutures create an air-tight seal around the obturator.

- Once the deepest facial layer is divided, attach a Littlewoods forceps to it at each end of the incision.
- The assistant should pull each Littlewoods forceps up at right angles to the abdomen to tent the abdominal wall off the underlying peritoneal contents.
- Clear the preperitoneal fat from the peritoneum with a sucker.
- Tent the peritoneum up with a Littlewoods forceps and open with scissors to gain entry to the peritoneal cavity (Figure 25.1).
- Select an appropriately long port that is also wide enough to accommodate the extraction bag at the end of the procedure. Place this directly through the peritoneal incision using a blunt obturator.
- Use a 2/0 suture to purse-string around the port in two layers (the peritoneal layer plus at least one fascial layer) to create an air-tight seal (Figure 25.2).
- Insufflate and check port placement with the laparoscope.

26

A modification to the Hassan technique for securing pneumoperitoneum

Ben Challacombe and Pardeep Kumar

Initial port insertion is a key step in minimally invasive surgery. It should be done safely and quickly, leaving an air-tight seal. The umbilicus is a common choice for camera port insertion for pelvic surgery. A 1–2 cm skin incision is made superior to the umbilicus. A Littlewoods forceps is then used to develop the space either side of the umbilical stalk which is then grasped and lifted. An 11 blade is then inserted to create a 5 mm incision at the junction of the umbilical stalk and rectus sheath (Figures 26.1 and 26.2). Curved Mayo scissors are then inserted (concave surface facing up) with steady pressure whilst lifting the stalk until a pop is felt as the scissor tips enter the peritoneal cavity. A downward angle is required during this manoeuvre otherwise the scissors simply travel into the space of Retzius. The scissors are then opened slightly once in the peritoneal cavity and withdrawn in the open position (to avoid bowel injury) to widen the fascial defect (Figures 26.3 and 26.4). A finger sweep can then be conducted in the normal manner and the port inserted and secured as per individual preference.

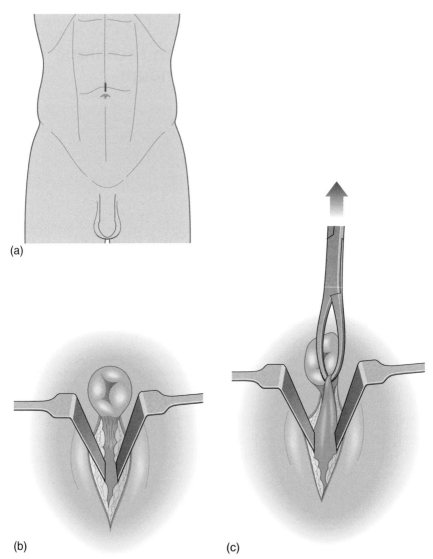

Figure 26.1 (a) Midline 2 cm incision down to the anterior rectus sheath. Caudal limit circatrix. (b) Retract skin and subcutaneous fat laterally. Develop spaces lateral to the umbilical stalk with a Spencer Wells. Once the demarcation between stalk and sheath is well delineated, grasp the stalk and lift at right angles to the abdominal wall with the Spencer Wells. Upward traction to lift the abdominal wall away from the bowel should be maintained throughout the following steps. (c) With the stalk held up at tension, a full-thickness incision is made in the stalk to expose preperitoneal fat with 11 blade.

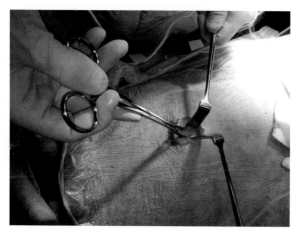

Figure 26.2 Gaining access to the peritoneum.

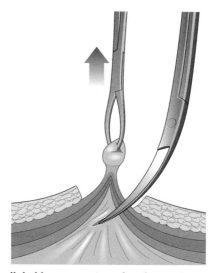

Figure 26.3 With the stalk held up at tension, closed curved Mayo scissors are introduced (concavity upwards) into the stalk incision and used to puncture the parietal peritoneum. The scissors are slowly withdrawn, slightly open, to increase the size of the peritoneal entry in one movement. Scissors are never reintroduced open. Stay sutures may be taken either side of the defect at the surgeon's preference. A finger sweep is performed and the initial port is inserted and secured. A single suture may be used to close the skin around the port if necessary.

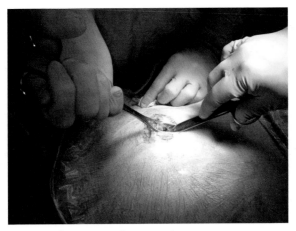

Figure 26.4 Scissors used to open and enter peritoneum.

27

Finger access is the safest

Richard Napier-Hemy

Speedy and safe access to the peritoneum can be gained with the index finger (or, when you develop the muscles, the little finger).

A standard lap primary port incision at the lateral border of the rectus abdominis is made. The index finger dissects through to the external oblique, clearing fat and Scarpa's fascia. Two Langenbeck retractors then hold the wound open and a 5–10 mm nick is made in the external oblique aponeurosis. The finger can then dissect through the rest of the muscle layers and the peritoneum without risk of sharp injury to bowel. An index finger will mean that a standard 12 mm port may leak so a balloon port such as the Covidien Blunt Tip Trocar (Figure 27.1) is useful. The little finger can gain access through a 10 mm incision which can be ideal for pyeloplasty where no tissue is to be removed.

This method is quicker than a standard Hassan's and so far has been safe in over 100 cases.

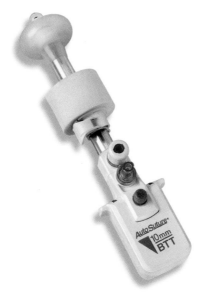

Figure 27.1 The Covidien Blunt Tip Trocar. (Copyright © 2012 Covidien. All rights reserved. Used with permission of Covidien.)

28

Keep it simple

Jon Cartledge

Patient position for renal laparoscopy

It is all too easy to focus on the complexities of surgical procedures but if a little time is taken to get the basics right then everything that follows will be much simpler.

Positioning a patient is made easy and safe by investment in a full body bean bag (Figure 28.1). The patient is placed in a comfortable lateral sleep position on a flat, unbroken table on top of a trauma-style bean bag. The bean bag should be flush with the table on the patient's front and hanging over the

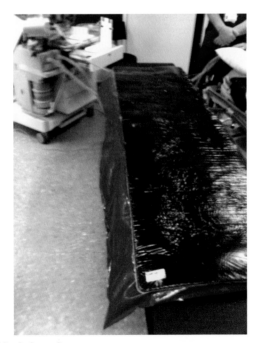

Figure 28.1 Full body bean bag.

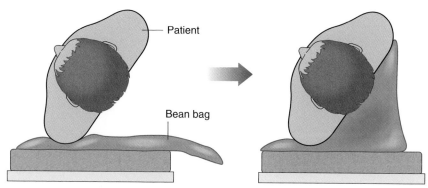

Figure 28.2 Full body bean bag is used to mould around patient.

edge of the table on their back. The patient is laid on their side, surgical side upwards and tilted slightly to the rear. Both arms are flexed and placed palm to palm level with the face. There is no need for a trough. The lower leg is bent and a pillow placed between the legs to support the straight upper leg. Ensure that there is no pillow protruding anterior to the thighs since this can impede the surgeon's hands. The bean bag is then moulded around the patient and the air removed (Figure 28.2). The bag stiffens and supports the patient. A single strap around the thigh holds the patient safely on the table, allowing lateral tilting with no need for additional support.

Port position for renal laparoscopy

Patients come in all shapes and sizes but the positioning of the three primary ports required for renal laparoscopy can be simplified using fixed landmarks.

The 10mm camera port is placed first following a Hassan cutdown but importantly, the position of this port should depend upon where the other operating ports are placed.

The iliac fossa port (Figure 28.3) (1) is the first fixed point and should be sited three fingers superomedial to the anterior superior iliac spine (ASIS). The superior port (2) will be placed in the midclavicular line just inferior to the costal margin. Only after these landmarks are noted should the position of the camera port be chosen at the third corner of the triangle (3). In this way the operating position and camera view will be optimal regardless of the patient's size and shape.

The correct plane

The most important step in transperitoneal renal laparoscopic surgery is identification of the plane between the posterior surface of the mesocolon and the anterior surface of Gerota's fascia (Figure 28.4). If this plane is identified cleanly then the rest of the procedure is straightforward.

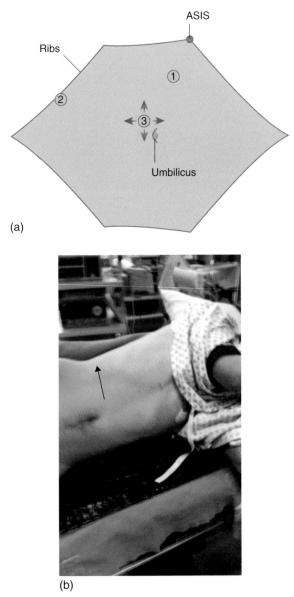

Figure 28.3 (a) Position of first, second and third ports. ASIS, anterior superior iliac spine. Dot below and to the right of number 3 indicates the umbilicus. (b) The ribs can be seen, as can the ASIS (arrow pointing at pelvic area).

The first step is to incise the reflection of the peritoneum lateral to the colon. Care should be taken to ensure that only this thin layer is incised so that the filmy fascia overlying the fat covering the posterior abdominal wall is not breached.

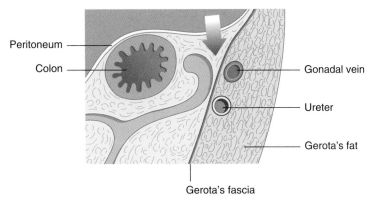

Peritoneum

Colon

Gonadal vein

Ureter

Gerota's fat

Gerota's fascia

Figure 28.4 Entry plane in between the posterior surface of the mesocolon and the anterior surface of Gerota's fascia

The colon is reflected medially. It may be necessary to retract the fat posterior to this in a lateral direction. It is crucial not to tear the filmy fascia overlying this fat. This plane of dissection is developed following the fascia medially (downwards on the surgical monitor) until a horizontal transition is seen in the fat layer. Close inspection will reveal that there is a clear edge here – the lateral most reflection of the mesocolon. That mesocolon must be drawn forward whilst preserving the filmy fascia that is overlying Gerota's fascia at this point. If this dissection is done level with the lower pole of the kidney, the next structures encountered will be the gonadal vein and ureter showing behind the filmy fascia. Only now should Gerota's fascia be incised to expose the ureter and vein.

29

The Ten Commandments

Peter Rimmington

1 *First, get everything ready*. Get all your instruments set up, check they are all in theatre and working, do a white balance, etc., before you start cutting for the first port site.
2 *Port placement is everything*. To make an easy operation difficult, put your ports in the wrong place. THINK … where is my target organ, and how am I approaching it? Laparoscopy is for thinking surgeons.
3 *Countertraction shows the planes*. Keep left- and right-hand instruments working close together as this aids vision and allows the gas to help show the surgical planes. The question I ask trainees the most during surgery is 'What is your left hand doing?'. Usually nothing! Declan Cahill always says, 'The tissues are not stuck down! You are in the wrong plane!'.
4 *Dissect enough for anatomical certainty*. If you are not sure where that vessel goes or what it serves, dissect until you are sure. Never clip, tie or cut until you are sure.
5 *Do NOT work down a tunnel*. Approach your target area on a wide front. If you work down an ever narrowing tunnel and there is bleeding, the tunnel will always fill faster than you can suck. A broad approach lets the blood run away from the area and you can pinpoint it and deal with it.
6 *Blood is the enemy of vision*. The only acceptable blood loss is zero blood loss! There are a plethora of effective dissection tools available so that cold scissor cutting or generous 'sweeping' of tissue (also known as crow barring) is unnecessary! Every bit of bleeding mounts up until you have a black background to your field and need to insert swabs to boost the available light.
7 *Use the correct tool for the job*. If you asked me to come and help you change a car tyre and I arrived with a fire extinguisher, you would think I was a nutter! So use a right angle to clear vessels, use needle holders to hold needles, etc. The reason people don't always do this is lack of proprioception to reinsert the new instrument to the same place they were working. This means you need more box practice.

8 *Think 'what is on the other side?'.* Most inadvertent injuries are caused by heat transfer or forceful dissection. Always think, what is on the other side of this tissue? Duodenum on the right renal hilum, pancreas/spleen/bowel on the left. So be gentle and avoid heat if possible.

9 *Check haemostasis at low pressure.* Before closing and extracting the specimen, drop the pressure to 6 mmHg and look for venous bleeding. Also check the ports for bleeding at this time. This is now a medicolegal requirement so document it in the notes as well!

10 *The bag works like a scoop.* Don't try to stuff the specimen into the bag; it will break. Lift the specimen up, put the bag underneath and drop the specimen into the bag or scoop it up like you would a fish into a net.

Print out these Ten Commandments, laminate them and hang them on your 'stack'. If you are struggling with a case, run through them and I am sure they will help.

30

Controlling a small hole in the inferior vena cava

Richard Napier-Hemy

A small hole in the inferior vena cava (IVC) does not always need to be sutured or converted to open surgery. In this case, the right gonadal vein was avulsed during mobilisation of the pelvoureteral junction (PUJ) before a pyeloplasty. The bleeding could be controlled with one Johannes forceps through a low port. A further port was placed cranial to the defect and the IVC controlled by pinching above and below the site of the gonadal vein. The 5 mm hole was then clipped with a sequence of Ligaclips. No single clip went the whole way across the defect, but four clips managed to completely control the bleeding with no need for conversion and more rapid control than suturing.

See Figures 30.1 and 30.2.

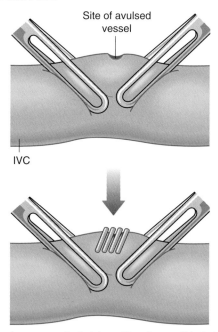

Figure 30.1 Johannes forceps applied either side of a small hole in the cava and clips applied.

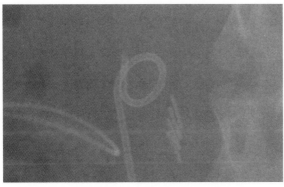

Figure 30.2 Postoperative radiology showing clips and a drain.

31

Remember Endoloops?

Richard Napier-Hemy

Endoloop Vicryl self-knotting loops (Ethicon) are commonly used by general surgeons for appendicectomies. They can be very useful in urology as well.

- For transvesical control of the lower ureter via a suprapubic stab into the bladder, the ureteric orifice can be mobilised with instruments inserted via a nephroscope urethrally or by using a grasping forceps and Collings knife. The ureter can then be occluded by looping the Endoloop over the ureter and grasping the ureter with transurethral forceps. The Endoloop can then be snugged down to occlude the ureter before nephroureterectomy.
- Very large ureters cannot be closed using conventional clips. The Endoloop is useful for this.
- Control of a short stump of a vessel: if the vessel has only one clip on it and probably needs a further clip for safest control, but is too short to be grasped and delivered for clipping, an Endoloop placed around graspers holding onto the vessel can be deployed around the vessel (Figure 31.1).

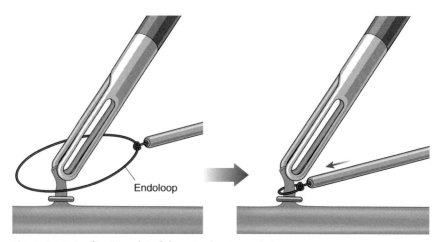

Figure 31.1 Application of Endoloop to short vessel stump.

32

Tips in laparoscopic urology

Dominic Hodgson

Preparation

Chris Eden advised me to shave with my non-dominant hand to develop ambidexterity, and I now find it difficult to shave with my right!

It's inexcusable to substitute practice in a wet or dry lab for practice on your patients. Regarding practice in suturing, all you need is a pair of needle holders, a shoe box, some sutures, an eye-patch and a balloon dismembered and secured with drawing pins. Put the lid on the box, having cut a square hole in the final third and poke the instruments through the lid somewhere near the edge of the hole.

Conversion

Timely conversion is a sign of strength, not weakness. Conversion rates for stone nephrectomies will inevitably be higher than for radical nephrectomies. Don't beat yourself up about conversion: the dissection that you have achieved before opening will have been less morbid than if it had been an open procedure from the start and the incision will probably be smaller.

To get an idea of how difficult a radical nephrectomy will be and how big a hole you might have to make, look not at the pole-to-pole parenchymal length but the intra-Gerota's fascia length, which accounts for fat, on the preoperative computed tomograph (CT).

Bleeding

I always drop the pressure to 4 mmHg at the end of a case to check for venous bleeding. I'm sure that this has prevented me returning to theatre on at least one occasion.

Instruments

The 10 mm right-angled dissector is a great instrument for nephrectomies. It may be that you use an extra 10 mm rather than a 5 mm port to accommodate it, but that's not such a big deal. The instrument is excellent for preparing vessels, the renal vein especially so.

Pyeloplasty

I don't think there is a major advantage for a trans- or retroperitoneal approach. Some say it's better to have a retroperitoneal leak but if that is happening you probably need to go back to the dry lab to practise suturing.

Unless you have preoperative contrast imaging of the ureter, I would recommend a retrograde study, especially in the elderly, to rule out a malignant cause for obstruction or a distal stricture. And if you put your stent in at this stage, use a 28 cm × 4.8 F one; you are less likely to subsequently cut it and it's easier to suture around.

You should partially transect the ureter and spatulate but don't fully dismember until you have your heal stitch in.

33

Laparoscopic suturing using the Storz dolphin-nosed forceps

Alan McNeill

I think my best tip relates to laparoscopic suturing at laparoscopic prostatectomy. I tend to open the jaws of the needle holder to assist throwing the knot (Figure 33.1).

Note:

1 Use of a Storz dolphin-nosed forceps in the left hand.
2 Needle holder used in right hand.
3 Jaws of needle holder opened towards instrument in left hand to make throw easier.

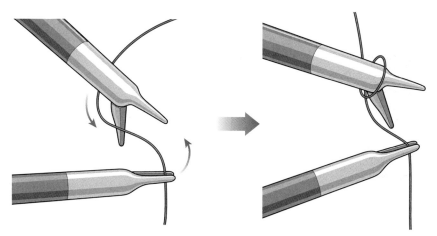

Figure 33.1 Opening the jaws of the needle holder to assist throwing the knot.

34

Laparoscopic suturing

Henry Sells

When carrying out laparoscopic suturing, it can be tiring to use a laparoscopic needle holder if holding it the same way as you would hold a tennis racket handle, particularly if, like me, you are a short surgeon. Holding the laparoscopic needle holder like a pen takes a bit of getting used to but it is less tiring on the shoulder and I think gives more subtle control of the instrument. It can be more difficult to release the ratchet but this is something the surgeon gets used to.

35

Improving your laparoscopic suturing

Chris Eden

When suturing laparoscopically, you should always use two needle holders and insert the needle on a needle holder with the hand with which you want to suture. Once the needle is inside the patient, you should loosely grasp the tip of the needle and rotate it if necessary to mount it correctly using the opposite needle holder.

The needle should be passed through tissues using rotation rather than pushing and should be removed from tissues again by rotation. No more than a centimetre of tail should be left before throwing knots.

For ease of throwing the knots, it is sensible to use the curve of the needle to hold the suture material away from the needle holder in a horizontal direction and to use the same knotting sequence each time. I use two clockwise throws followed by one anti-clockwise throw and finish with two clockwise throws. The thread should then be cut relatively short in order not to confuse the cut ends of the tail with the next suture.

36

Cholangiogram catheters can help antegrade wire placement at the time of pyeloplasty

Richard Napier-Hemy

Many surgeons place JJ stents antegradely during laparoscopic pyeloplasty. Conventionally, a wire is placed via a Venflon into the peritoneum and then manipulated into the ureter. Often, one grasper is holding on to the ureter and the other holds the wire, but there is no free hand to easily feed the wire down the ureter. A cholangiogram catheter is a 15 cm long cannula with an angled tip (Figure 36.1). This can be placed directly into the upper ureter and the wire advanced down easily without the need for an extra hand.

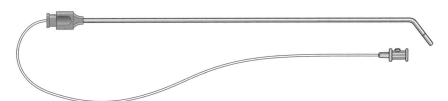

Figure 36.1 Horner's cholangiogram catheter by Steriseal.

37

Laparoscopic nephrectomy: introduction of a balloon-tipped trocar in an obese patient

Damian Hanbury

A big (3–4 cm) skin incision makes your cutdown to the rectus sheath much easier and allows decent retraction. Recess the gauze collar of the balloon-tipped trocar down to the rectus sheath to keep an air-tight seal.

See Figure 37.1.

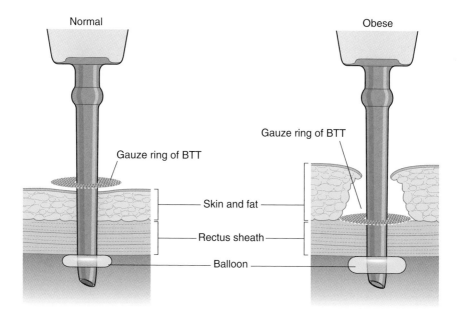

Figure 37.1 Using the balloon-tipped trocar.

38

Laparoscopic nephrectomy: closing the exit site in an obese patient

Damian Hanbury

Closing the muscle layers of a deep specimen exit site in an obese patient is a real challenge. The trick is to site the figure-of-eight sutures using a J needle. Clip and cut the sutures and leave them loose. This way your exposure is maximised for the whole closure. Only pull up and tie when all sutures are positioned. Repeat for each layer.

See Figure 38.1.

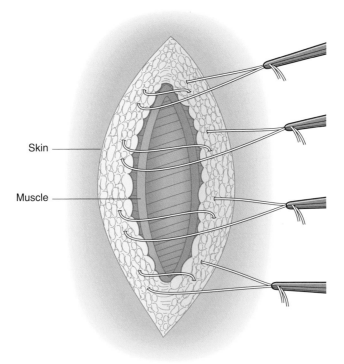

Figure 38.1 Multiple clips used to stay sutures so they can all be positioned before tying.

39

Laparoscopic nephrectomy: port sites for left nephrectomy

Damian Hanbury

In Figure 39.1:
- port A is inserted at the intersection of the lateral border of the rectus sheath and costal margin
- port B at the intersection of the lateral border of the rectus sheath and a line running from the umbilicus to the anterior superior iliac spine (ASIS)
- C is the 'optic port' for insertion of the camera. Appropriate triangulation between A and B, slightly nearer the upper port site.

Remember to mark before picking up the knife!

For right nephrectomy, use a mirror image and employ an additional port for liver retraction.

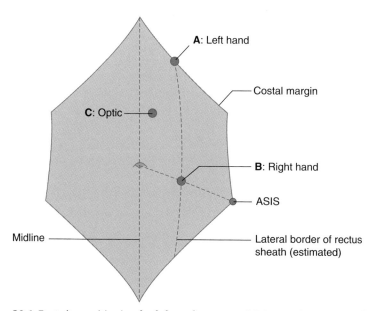

Figure 39.1 Port site positioning for left nephrectomy. ASIS, anterior superior iliac spine. Optic refers to port for camera.

40

Laparoscopic nephrectomy

Peter W. Cooke

During laparoscopic nephrectomy, if you are anticipating bleeding or a difficult area of dissection, put small swabs in before you start. Open them right up and keep out of field of view (they reflect the light and close the camera iris, making the view dark). They are then ready for gaining control and maintaining view immediately. Versaports can be unscrewed to allow removal. Don't forget to remove.

For retroperitoneal nephrectomy, use four ports and put a large fan retractor through the middle one of your three working ports, attached to a flexible instrument holder. I use the 'Flex-arm'. This bolts to the table and allows you to lift the kidney and fix it, putting the hilum on stretch and, most importantly, enables you to use both hands to perform the hilar dissection, beneath the fan retractor (like a pit prop holding up the roof in a coal mine). This is much easier than retracting the kidney with one hand and dissecting single-handedly with the other. Readjust it as the hilar dissection proceeds to keep vessels on maximal traction. If the renal vein is too broad for a Weck Hem-o-Lok clip, tie with a Vicryl suture to narrow it, and then clip it. Ensure that the scrub nurse knows which way to mount the Weck in the applicator to ensure they are parallel to each other, and to the inferior vena cava or aorta.

41

Employing an extra port for laparoscopic nephrectomy

Toby Page

When performing left laparoscopic nephrectomy, especially in the patient with an increased Body Mass Index (BMI), have no hesitation in inserting an extra 5 mm port 1–2 cm anterior to the midaxillary line, usually just superior to the level of the camera port. This can be used to help with splenic dissection without being at the limit of the instruments, so giving better control. It can also be used by the camera holder or another assistant both to retract the colon medially and to help with kidney retraction. At the end of the procedure, if a drain is going to be left, it can be inserted through this extra port which is usually a comfortable position for the patient. If you feel you are stretching or struggling to reach the upper pole or splenic area, this extra port quickly and easily resolves the problem, allowing better instrument control and reducing instrument wobble. If you are thinking an extra port would help, stop thinking about it and put it in!

42

Improved control of the renal vein during laparoscopic nephrectomy

Tony Riddick

I sometimes use a Vicryl tie to snug down the renal vein before applying a Hem-o-Lok. The technique uses a 6 inch length doubled back and I use a right angle to pass it behind the vein, grasping the loop by the tip. Once the loop is passed round, use the grasper to grab the two free ends through the loop and this compresses the collapsed vein. It is then very easy to put on the Weck Hem-o-Lok clip.

43

Aiding dissection of the renal artery during a laparoscopic radical nephrectomy

Adam Jones

On the left side, a good way to aid exposure of the renal artery is to use the divided gonadal vein stump as a means of retracting the renal vein. Divide the gonadal vein between at least four clips on the stay side and two clips on the go side. These should be placed 3 cm from the junction with the renal vein so as not to interfere with the subsequent division of the renal vein. By pulling on the gonadal vein stump cranially, exposure to the renal artery is significantly improved. The multiple clips ensure that should a clip be accidentally pulled off by this traction, it is not really a problem.

44

Robotic-assisted laparoscopic pyeloplasty

Prokar Dasgupta

During Anderson-Hynes dismembered robotic-assisted laparoscopic pyelo-plasty (RALP), I suture the most dependent part of the reduced renal pelvis to the heel of the spatulated ureter using a 4/0 Vicryl suture 15 cm in length. The suture should be well greased. Unlike open pyeloplasty where the posterior anastomosis is completed first, I then use the same suture to stitch the anterior wall of the renal pelvis to the anterior wall of the spatulated ureter initially. This is the most accessible part of the anastomosis and allows the posterior wall to present itself during RALP. The suturing becomes rapid and the JJ stent does not get in the way of the instruments.

45

Laparoscopic prostatectomy

Peter W. Cooke

For lap prostatectomy, put a Clutton's sound in and get your nurse to push down to lengthen the urethra when working on the anterior apex. This makes more space for the dorsal vein complex (DVC) stitch and prevents the suture transfixing the urethra. It can be used to lift the prostate on bladder neck division/seminal vesicle dissection. It puts the urethra on stretch for easier dissection/urethral division at that point.

NB: It must be removed when doing posterior dissection towards the apex as it fixes the prostate and makes posterior dissection difficult.

When the prostate is dissected free, put in an Endo Catch bag via the most lateral left-hand port. Remove the port and pull the string to bring the bag just beneath the muscle. Reinsert the port alongside the bag (under vision so as not to split the bag).

At the end of the procedure, remove the port and pull the string into the abdomen via the right-hand port, replace the left-hand port, put the camera through the left-hand port and pull the bag string up to the midline camera port so the prostate can be extracted through the camera port incision, which is already a wider incision and is easily closed by suturing the anterior rectus sheath in one layer.

Stand on a box for any suturing as it's more comfortable on the shoulders.

Push the gas pressure up to 20 mmHg for apical dissection to minimise bleeding and give the best view. Do not suck any blood as it just makes it bleed more, by lowering pressure. Get your assistant to drip water from above the DVC to give clear view.

If there is any mild DVC/urethral bleeding after the prostate is dissected free, put in a catheter, blow up the balloon and get the scrub nurse to put on some traction to stop the bleeding while you use an Endo Catch bag or reconstruct the bladder neck, check for haemostasis around the bladder base, etc. Invariably any minor bleeding stops. Get on with the anastomosis and the bladder will snug down and stop any ooze, rather than using lots of diathermy or clips, etc., close to the anastomosis/sphincter.

46

Use of the Endo Close device for prostatic elevation during robotic-assisted radical prostatectomy

David Bouchier-Hayes

This technique was taught to me by Dinesh Agarwal, a remarkable surgical innovator, and popularised by Tony Costello's unit in Melbourne. During robotic prostatectomy, following division of the anterior bladder neck, the prostate is elevated in order to be able to appreciate the delineation of the posterior aspect of the bladder neck and to maintain this elevation to allow for countertraction when continuing towards the vasa and seminal vesicles. Many surgeons either have the assistant or robotic third arm do this. This means that the assistant port may no longer be available, there is an extra instrument in the pelvis and the third arm or assistant cannot be used for other manoeuvres. This technique utilises the very simple Endo Close device (Covidien) to allow for elevation of the bladder neck into the operative field.

Following division of the anterior bladder neck, the catheter is delivered towards the abdominal wall. The Endo Close device, loaded with a 2/0 suture, is passed through the abdominal wall by the assistant, close to the symphysis (Figure 46.1). The device is passed through the eye of the catheter, the suture is grasped and the device disengaged (Figures 46.2 and 46.3). The device is withdrawn through the eye of the catheter and the suture is re-engaged (Figure 46.4). The suture is then brought through the abdominal wall and fixed in place with an artery forceps. Countertraction

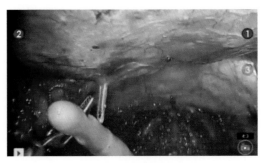

Figure 46.1 Bring up the catheter with the robotic arm.

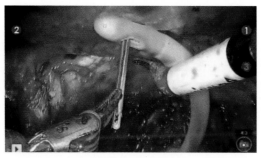

Figure 46.2 Insert the needle through the eye of the catheter.

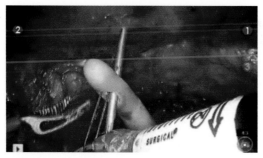

Figure 46.3 Needle being threaded through the eye of the catheter.

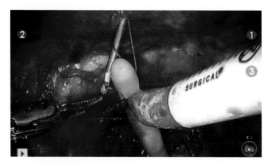

Figure 46.4 Suture re-engaged.

is applied at the penile end of the catheter, and another artery forceps is used to keep tension on the catheter, allowing for elevation of the prostate (Figure 46.5). The procedure itself takes no more than 30 sec to a minute, and is very inexpensive as the device can be reused to close the assistant port at the end of the case.

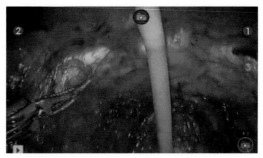

Figure 46.5 Tensioning the catheter.

47

Additional points of note when performing prostate suspension during minimally invasive radical prostatectomy

Ben Challacombe

If the Endo Close is not brought through the midline, bleeding may occur from the rectus abdominis muscle. If this occurs, complete the manoeuvre to tamponade the bleeding which usually stops. Use monofilament, not braided suture as it runs more easily in the abdominal wall.

When releasing the Endo Close to regrasp the suture on the other side of the catheter, move the catheter down rather than the Endo Close. This will avoid inadvertent removal of the Endo Close.

When placing the clip on the catheter at the external urethral meatus when providing countertraction, take care not to catch the glans penis or foreskin in the jaws.

48

Robotic radical prostatectomy

Senthil Nathan

When the fourth arm is required to dissect the seminal vesicle, a 2/0 Vicryl stitch can be passed through the median ligament of the bladder, which is then brought out through the 5 mm assistant port to continue the retraction while the seminal vesicles and the prostate are dissected off the rectum.

49

A technique to relocate the robotic prostatectomy retrieval bag to the midline camera port

Muhammad Jamal Khan and Omer Karim

During robotic-assisted laparoscopic prostatectomy, the prostatectomy specimen is collected in an Endo Catch bag, the silk suture of which exits the abdomen from a laterally placed 12 mm laparoscopic port. At the end of the procedure, the exit site of the silk suture needs to be moved to retrieve the specimen through the midline incision. We describe a simple method to relocate the silk suture to a different exit wound in a controlled manner rather than blindly 'winkling' a finger in the abdomen to catch the silk suture and pull it through the midline incision.

At the end of the procedure following undocking of the surgical da Vinci robot, the camera port is removed and an index finger inserted via this wound into the abdominal cavity to identify the end of the laterally placed 12 mm port. The port is completely occluded with the tip of the finger. The laparoscopic sucker is inserted via the 12 mm port and pushed against the tip of the finger while the finger retreats and guides the tip of the sucker out of the midline incision. The tips of the laparoscopic needle holders are then inserted into the hollow end of the sucker tip and used to push the sucker back out of the 12 mm port. The end of the specimen bag silk suture is then grasped in the laparoscopic needle holders which are then pulled back through the midline incision, together with the silk suture (Figure 49.1). This incision may then be enlarged to allow delivery of the specimen bag.

The technique may be adapted for other laparoscopic procedures.

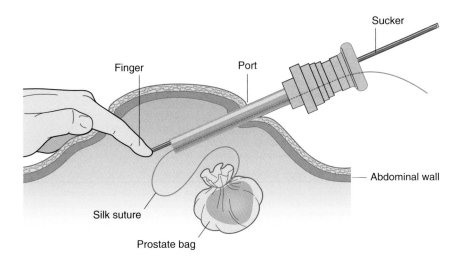

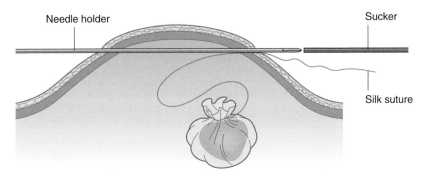

Figure 49.1 Laparoscopic sucker in use.

50

The rectal injury test

Ben Challacombe

Rectal injury is a devastating complication of minimally invasive pelvic surgery (prostatectomy and cystectomy). However, it can be dealt with easily if recognised intraoperatively with minimal additional morbidity to the patient. We routinely carry out a rectal test in all patients who have a wide local excision, salvage surgery, inflamed/adherent posterior planes and those where we suspect a rectal injury could occur. This is done in the following manner.

1 Initial digital rectal examination to check for obvious rectal laceration or blood on the gloved finger.
2 Insertion of the rectal tube past the dentate line.
3 Insufflation of the rectum with 50 cc of air using a 50 mL syringe with catheter tip.
4 Deflation of the rectum and filling of the pelvis with irrigant (usually normal saline).
5 Insufflation of the rectum with 100 cc air and observation for bubbles. If these are present, slowly aspirate irrigant and follow the bubbles to the site of rectal injury if this isn't obvious.
6 Repair as appropriate +/− covering stoma (not usually needed in cases where injury is recognised intraoperatively). If an injury is suspected in the postoperative period, a water-soluble enema is the best investigation.

51

Identifying potential breaches in the rectum during minimally invasive surgery

Justin Collins

As more salvage prostatectomies are being undertaken, the incidence of rectal perforation is increasing. There are various ways to check for a rectal perforation such as digital rectal examination (DRE) and checking the glove for blood or obvious hole seen during surgery. Another approach is to fill the pelvis with irrigation fluid and watch for air bubbles.

If you are doing robotic or laparoscopic prostatectomy, you can also gently insert a clear plastic proctoscope and insert a cystoscope with light source down the inside of the proctoscope. The light source to the camera of the robot or laparoscope can then be turned off and this will result in illumination of the rectum. It will then be evident if there are breaches and also areas of thinning that need to be oversewn, thereby also identifying potential breaches in the rectum.

52

The wrong plane

Anonymous

I have often heard it said that 'When performing laparoscopic radical prostatectomy, if you find the tissues very stuck, they are not stuck at all. You are in the wrong plane!'. This brilliant but simple tip has served me well. I think it originally came from Declan Cahill.

We are now entering an era of post-template prostatectomies and I hope this observation will continue to hold true.

53

Spreading tough tissue with robotic forceps

Marc Laniado

Applying Weck clips requires that the ends of the clip meet to close, otherwise they will fall off. Robotic forceps can be used to spread tissues to make a space in which the tips of the clips can meet. When pushing forceps through tissues, the forceps may not be able to spread wide enough because the tissues are too tough. This is commonly the case when trying to place clips to tie off the vascular pedicle during a robotic prostatectomy.

I learned the following trick watching Randy Fagin. When the forceps have passed through the tissues and have opened a little, there is usually enough space to insert the tips of the robotic scissors through the open forceps. By spreading the scissors inside the forceps, it is usually possible to generate enough force to spread the tissues adequately. A space is then made for the Weck to be placed securely.

54

Robotic-assisted radical prostatectomy

Prokar Dasgupta

During robotic-assisted radical prostatectomy (RARP), I open the endopelvic fascia although I am aware that some colleagues do not. My reasoning is that nearly half my patients have palpable disease and therefore opening the fascia allows me good posterior access and wide excision or incremental nerve sparing should that be necessary. I am careful to touch the urethra as little as possible and avoid aggressive dissection lateral to the dorsal vein complex (DVC) after opening the endopelvic fascia. This preserves the pelvic floor and sphincteric support and allows early return of continence. In order to precisely identify the junction between the DVC and urethra during RARP, I request my assistant to gently pull on the urethral catheter. This identifies the groove between the two structures and thus allows a DV stitch to be inserted at that point. If this suture is placed in the right place, bleeding from the DVC when cut is minimal.

55

Steps to free up robotic arm and assistant availability during robotic radical prostatectomy

Adam Jones

Exposure is everything. We use a couple of steps that maintain exposure without tying up a robotic arm or assistant. Firstly, after dividing the anterior bladder neck, we reposition the catheter so it comes out through the open anterior bladder neck. A Carter Thomason needle holding a 30 cm length of 0 Prolene at its midpoint is inserted under direct vision as close to the symphysis pubis as possible in the midline. The needle is threaded directly through the distal eyeholes of the catheter and the loop of Prolene suture held by a robotic grasper. The Carter Thomason needle is then withdrawn from the catheter eyeholes but maintained in the abdomen. The Prolene midpoint is then grasped again from the robotic grasper by the Carter Thomason needle and withdrawn from the abdomen. This end is pulled up and secured with an artery clip flush with the skin. This pulls the catheter to the anterior abdominal wall. The 'bag' end of the catheter is then pulled backwards from the penis. The catheter is secured in position using a protective gauze swab and a Roberts clamp to maintain the catheter at retraction. This elevates the prostate, allowing easy division of the posterior bladder neck and access to the vasa and seminal vesicles without needing to use either robotic arm or an assistant, allowing both to provide exposure elsewhere.

Once mobilised, the seminal vesicles and vasa are usually elevated by a robotic arm and/or an assistant to allow access to Denonvillier's fascia. By placing a suture robotically through the anterior abdominal wall and then through the seminal vesicles and vasa before returning to the anterior abdominal wall and tying, the seminal vesicle/vasa complex can be elevated and held out of the way.

Typically the prostate will be entrapped in an Endo Catch bag inserted through the assistant 12 mm port. This port is also used to introduce the needles for subsequent anastomosis. There is a risk that the Endo Catch bag thread and the sutures could become entangled. To avoid this, we reinsert the Endo Catch bag thread into the abdomen after closing the bag and then withdraw this thread from the 5 mm suction port.

56

Use of Ethicon Vicryl foil and robotic camera lights to warm the robotic scope lens to prevent lens fogging

Muhammad Jamal Khan and Omer Karim

Condensation on the scope lens resulting from differences between room and intra-abdominal temperature is a disturbing problem for laparoscopic surgeons. We report a simple, cheap and effective method for preventing lens condensation by lens heating using the Ethicon Vicryl foil and robotic camera lights (Figure 56.1).

As shown in Figure 56.1, the robotic scope tip is kept in Ethicon Vicryl foil (W9377). The camera lights switch on to full. There is an abrupt rise in temperature at the tip of the scope (as measured by thermometer). Within 60 sec, the temperature reaches 38 °C. In 2 min it reaches 40 °C and in 3 min 41 °C.

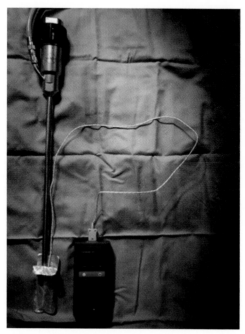

Figure 56.1 Robotic camera lights, foil and thermometer.

57

Management of anastomotic leak following radical prostatectomy

Ruzi Begum and Omer Karim

Vesicourethral anastomotic leak can be a devastating complication of radical prostate surgery. A modified catheter with a second drainage hole proximal to the balloon corresponding to the level of the anastomosis is useful in these cases. This enables drainage from both the level of the anastomosis and from within the bladder, resulting in rapid cessation of any anastomotic leak. This type of catheter is available commercially but can also be fashioned from a standard Foley catheter and should be the catheter of choice for a radical prostatectomy (Figure 57.1).

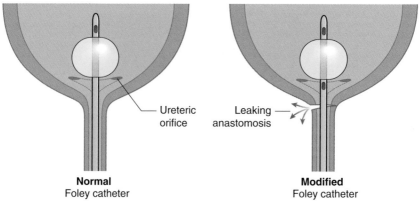

Ureteric orifice	Leaking anastomosis
Normal Foley catheter	**Modified** Foley catheter

Figure 57.1 Modified Foley catheter.

58

Identification of ureters during minimally invasive radical cystectomy

Ben Challacombe

Many surgeons construct the urinary diversion through a small abdominal incision in an extracorporeal manner after laparoscopic or robotic-assisted radical cystectomy. We describe a simple technique to facilitate identification of the ureters. When mobilising the distal ureter at the bladder, two large Weck Hem-o-Lok clips are applied prior to division. By securing a 0 Vicryl tie to the proximal Weck clip and leaving the proximal end of the tie in the paracolic gutter, the ureters may be easily identified when the patient is opened. A modification of this is to bring the proximal ties out through one of the ports towards the end of the procedure. The left-hand tie may also be used to facilitate transposition of the left ureter to the right side under the mesentery of the sigmoid colon in front of the sacral promontory.

59

Maintaining pneumoperitoneum during minimally invasive female cystectomy

Ben Challacombe

Opening of the vagina during female cystectomy is a necessary step which can cause problems during minimally invasive surgery as the loss of insufflation pressure compromises vision and working space as gas escapes through the introitus. The use of a 30×30 cm swab wrapped around a sponge forceps can help maintain this pressure. Manipulation of the forceps can also help facilitate vaginal sparing surgery. Placing the swab inside a green glove enables early identification of the vaginal lumen during dissection.

60

Robotic-assisted radical cystectomy

Prokar Dasgupta

I insert a disposable sigmoidoscope into the rectum preoperatively and strap it to the patient's thighs. During robotic-assisted radical cystectomy (RARC) the dissection is 'below, up' rather than 'above, down'. One of the first steps is posterior dissection between the rectum and bladder/prostate. In bulky tumours the up-and-down movement of the sigmoidoscope allows identification of the rectum and reduces the risk of rectal injury. I learnt this trick from Peter Rimington at Eastbourne during laparoscopic radical cystectomy. Another trick is to use a rectal balloon that can be intermittently inflated to show the rectum. This one was passed on to me by Khurshid Guru from New York.

While nerve sparing during RARC can be performed just as well as during robotic prostatectomy, it is important to remember that this step begins higher up during cystectomy. Aggressive dissection in the presacral space and at the tips of the seminal vesicles may render subsequent nerve sparing behind the prostate useless.

PART 3
Upper Tract Endourology

Top Tips in Urology, Second Edition. Edited by John McLoughlin, Neil Burgess,
Hanif Motiwala, Mark J. Speakman, Andrew Doble and John D. Kelly.
© 2013 John Wiley & Sons, Ltd. Published 2013 by John Wiley & Sons, Ltd.

61

Puncturing the calyx in order to obtain access for percutaneous nephrolithotomy: the three-finger rule

Gerald Rix

This was shown to me by Sammi Moussa in Edinburgh. I perform percutaneous nephrolithotomy (PCNL) access with the patient prone. The needle is inserted through the skin at the level of the posterior axillary line and angled so that it runs towards the calyx you are going to target. The C-arm of the image intensifier is placed at 0° in an anteroposterior (AP) setting for this. What you don't know is whether you are too high, i.e. above the calyx, or too deep and have gone beyond it.

Once you have passed the needle and it is lying apparently within the collecting system, you rotate the C-arm by 5° either away from the operating surgeon or towards the operating surgeon. When you take a flash again, if the needle is too high then it will appear to jump laterally if you move the image intensifier to the left 5° or medially if you rotate the image intensifier to the right by 5°. Equally, if the needle is too deep then by moving the C-arm 5° to the left, the needle will appear to jump to the left and by moving the C-arm 5° to the right, it will appear to jump to the right in relation to the calyx. If it doesn't move at all then it is in the right place. If the needle is too deep or too high, return the C-arm to the neutral position and whilst maintaining exactly the same AP plane, pull it out and then reinsert it at the correct depth. Then repeat the 5° shift of the C-arm to see if it is now lying in the correct place.

The way to remember this is by using three fingers of your own hand (use the left hand if operating on the left kidney and the right hand if operating on the right kidney). Hold all the fingers perpendicular to the floor and look down on them with one eye closed. Your eye is now doing what the C-arm does. If you watch the relationship of the three fingers to each other, you will see that relative to the middle finger, your index finger moves to the right if you look to the left (this is equivalent to a needle that is too high) whilst the ring finger (which is equivalent to a needle that is too deep) moves to the left. Equally, if you move your head or your eye to the right by 5°, the index finger tip appears to move to the left while the ring finger tip appears to move to the right.

I find that this method is easier than the bull's eye method of puncturing a calyx because it doesn't require so much manoeuvring of the C-arm.

62

Prevention of migration of the Amplatz sheath during percutaneous nephrolithotomy

Oliver Wiseman

During percutaneous nephrolithotomy (PCNL) in obese patients, there is a concern that the Amplatz sheath may not protrude sufficiently, and may migrate so that it is no longer retrievable.

The tying of two or three silk sutures as shown in Figures 62.1 and 62.2 will allow easy retrieval of the sheath should migration occur.

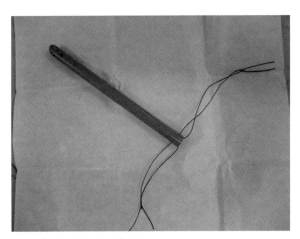

Figure 62.1 Sutures in place in Amplatz.

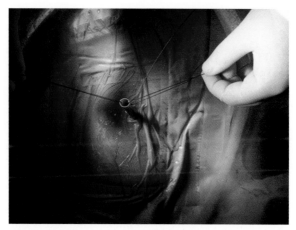

Figure 62.2 Sutures allow Amplatz to be pulled back.

63

Using safety wires during percutaneous nephrolithotomy

Sunil Kumar

It is important to ensure that once preliminary renal access is achieved prior to tract dilation by either the urologist or the radiologist, a serious attempt is made to ensure that a guidewire is passed down the ureter into the bladder. This should be confirmed on fluoroscopy with contrast. This can be a slippery wire initially, particularly if there is obstruction at the pelviureteric junction, but then would need to be replaced with an extra stiff wire and can be clipped away once the tract has been created. This in essence is the safety wire and helps to ensure that when the tract is created, other organs are not accidentally breached as we have all heard nightmare stories of access into the inferior vena cava (IVC), etc. If the sheath slips out accidentally during the procedure, the safety wire can guide you back into the pelvicalyceal system.

If the safety wire is lost accidentally during the procedure but access into the system is still present, another tip is to pass another wire up the open-ended ureteric catheter. This wire can now be grabbed under direct vision with the nephroscope in the renal pelvis and brought out via the sheath and clipped. The wire should also be clipped at the bottom end to prevent it from slipping. This means that the patient has a wire that is clipped at both ends and this wire can be used to reaccess the system or insert a stent if required.

This little trick of cheese-wiring the patient was shown to me by Anthony Timoney in Bristol.

64

Tips to make percutaneous nephrolithotomy easier

Aasem Chaudry

Securing the percutaneous nephrolithotomy tract

Percutaneous nephrolithotomy (PCNL) is a procedure frequently performed to treat renal stones. While this procedure has been in vogue for over two decades, there remains a wide variation in the techniques used. The technique has developed over time and continues to be improved. Traditionally, it was performed in a prone or semi-prone position but recently supine PCNL has become popular. Regardless of the position used, securing the tract after the initial successful puncture of the collecting system until completion remains a challenge. Loss of the tract during the procedure can be quite frustrating and re-entry into the collecting system can be quite difficult and at times unsuccessful. The technique described minimises the chances of this happening.

The use of a through-and-through guidewire passed via the ureteric access catheter from below and brought out of the PCN tract through the Amplatz sheath wherever possible is the best way of avoiding this complication. The guidewire is secured at both ends using simple artery forceps and is kept in place until completion of the procedure. If the Amplatz sheath slips out of the collecting system, re-entry is fairly straightforward and atraumatic.

8F self-retaining nephrostomy tube for post-PCNL drainage

The options for post-PCNL drainage consist of:
• self-retaining small-bore nephrostomy tube
• balloon catheter (Foley catheter)
• large-bore re-entry catheter with or without ureteric stent
• multi-access U-loop drainage tube
• simple rubber drain.
In the UK, the third option is most commonly used. However, the self-retaining small-bore nephrostomy tube is proposed as the best option. We have used this technique in 120 cases to date and have experienced reduced

analgesia, earlier removal of nephrostomy tube, less urine leakage, earlier discharge and no increase in blood loss. This suggests that a large-bore nephrostomy tube does not provide clinically significant tamponade to the tract, as was traditionally believed. In cases where post-PCNL external drainage is to be provided, we recommend a 8F self-retaining nephrostomy tube as the preferred option in uncomplicated PCNL. Advantages are:

- less patient discomfort
- early removal
- less postremoval urine leakage
- earlier discharge.

Technique to remove the Amplatz sheath after placement of nephrostomy tube

Two parallel cuts are made in the sheath approximately 5 mm apart and 2 cm in length. A strong artery forceps is used to grasp the strip from the wall of the sheath. The artery forceps is then rotated clockwise until the whole length of the sheath is divided and slides out smoothly. A skin stitch is then applied to secure the nephrostomy tube safely.

Securing the Amplatz sheath in morbidly obese patients undergoing PCNL

There are a number of options available to secure the Amplatz sheath other than using an extra-long access sheath. The technique described is simple and safe. A no.1 silk suture on a curved cutting needle is used. The needle is passed 2 cm from the edge at two points 180° apart. An artery clip is placed to hold each of the sutures. The sheath can then be placed in the desired position through a standard small incision. The sutures are used to keep the sheath in the desired position and pull it out safely at the end of the procedure.

Balloon tamponade of nephrostomy tract

Bleeding during and after PCNL remains a concern in spite of the recent improvment in tract-making techniques. Excessive bleeding is at times encountered during or after the procedure. In cases where the bleeding vessel cannot be identified and/or there is failure of simple measures like renal compression, early employment of this technique effectively controls bleeding quickly, avoiding the need for blood transfusion. Once bleeding is recognised to be excessive, the balloon used to dilate the tract initially is quickly reinserted over the guidewire already in place and is carefully placed to cover the entire tract. In cases of telescopic dilation of the tract, a new balloon will be required. The balloon is inflated under fluoroscopic guidance up to a pressure of 10 atmospheric. It is left *in situ* along with the guidewire and the procedure is discontinued. The balloon is then gradually deflated, reducing the pressure by

2 atmospheric every 10 min. After deflation, the same guidewire is used to place a nephrostomy tube. Further management is determined by clinical need. It is, however, recommended not to reuse the same tract in case a further session of PCNL is required.

Percutaneous cystolithotomy (PCCL), an underutilised technique for large bladder stones

Patients with bladder stones greater than 3 cm are suitable for this procedure. Similar principles are employed as for PCNL. The procedure involves placing the patient in a gentle lithotomy position and performing a cystoscopy to confirm the presence of a large hard stone. Suprapubic puncture at a suitable location is performed, the guidewire passed into the bladder and the percutaneous tract dilated using telescopic dilators under direct vision and the Amplatz sheath is placed. The stone breaking is completed as in PCNL. The suprapubic catheter is placed prior to removal of the Amplatz sheath. Cystoscopy is carried out at the end to ensure complete clearance of stones. The patient is discharged the same day or kept overnight to allow any bleeding to stop. The suprapubic catheter is removed after 48 h by the district nurse.

The advantages of this procedure are:
- no urethral trauma
- can be performed as a day case
- the equipment is already available in most urology units.

65

Using multiple guidewires during percutaneous nephrolithotomy

Stephanie J. Symons

When planning access for percutaneous nephrolithotomy (PCNL), it is important that all possible tracts required are taken into consideration (Figure 65.1). Although a single tract is generally all that is required, if flexible instruments are available, this is not the case universally. Therefore, if a second or even third tract may be necessary, it is important that the safety wires for these are placed before any single tract dilation is undertaken. It is very difficult to gain secondary percutaneous access once one tract is in place

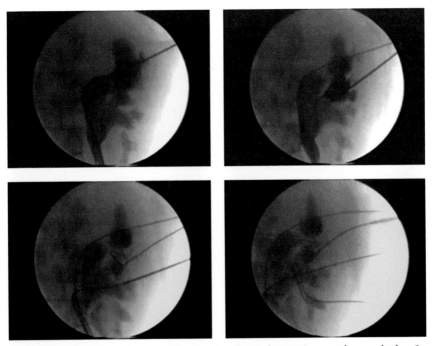

Figure 65.1 Placement of four guidewires for planned tracts in a staghorn calculus. In this case, no flexible instrument was available and a multi-tract PCNL was intended.

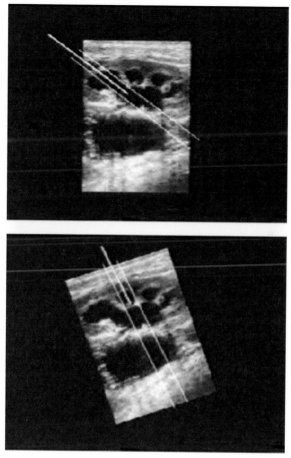

Figure 65.2 Correct and incorrect ultrasound images for 'calyceal puncture'.

due to cortical disruption and the subsequent inability to fill the collecting system satisfactorily. Any guidewires not required for subsequent tract dilation can be useful to highlight or even guide the nephroscope or flexible cystoscope/ureteroscope into a stone-laden calyx.

During ultrasound-guided percutaneous access, it is important that a straight tract from the calyceal cup to the renal pelvis is planned, just as for fluoroscopic access (Figure 65.2). Therefore, it is important to puncture the calyx only when the calyx, infundibulum and renal pelvis can be viewed in a straight line. This avoids unnecessary risk of perforation and bleeding during tract dilation and ensures the best movement for the nephroscope within the pelvicalyceal system.

66

Encrusted nephrostomy tubes

James Hall

This top tip is for removal of encrusted nephrostomy tubes/stents by placing the lithoclast probe along the offending tube and under fluoroscopy. The advised action is in fact more of a withdrawal of the tube over an actively oscillating lithoclast probe. Fluoroscopy is needed in case it goes through a side hole or perforates the tube.

This has saved us resorting to a PCNL a few times, most memorably in a nephrostomy tube stuck in a transplant kidney. When it is used for a stuck stent, it only tends to be possible in the female as the lower end of the stent needs to be outside the body to get the lithoclast probe in its lumen.

67

Reaching stones in the kidney during flexible ureterorenoscopy with a large renal pelvis

Gerald Rix

Sometimes stones, particularly in the lower pole, are very difficult to reach if there is a lot of space within the collecting system, even using a combination of active and passive deflection. You can see the stone but it is just out of reach of either the laser fibre or the basket. Under these circumstances, attaching a 10 mL syringe to the water channel will allow you to aspirate the collecting system which results in it shrinking down the space and often brings the stone right up to the tip of the scope.

68

The advantages of using the Peditrol during flexible and rigid ureterorenoscopy

Sunil Kumar

The Peditrol (Wismed, Durban, South Africa) is a device incorporating a foot pedal which delivers a dual flow (Figure 68.1). There is a continuous flow that can be regulated by altering the height of the irrigation fluid and there is also a bolus or accelerated flow that is regulated by a foot pedal which is under the control of the operating surgeon. The accelerated flow is produced on compressing the foot pedal and delivers a bolus of 3 mL of irrigation fluid. The speed of the foot compression regulates the amount of flow and once the foot pedal is released, the syringe refills automatically and is ready for a further bolus if required.

The advantages of the Peditrol are that it provides clear views that allow the surgeon to continue the procedure without needing to stop at regular intervals to allow the dust to settle. It also obviates the need for a runner in theatre whose responsibility is to control the pressure on the irrigating fluid. The Peditrol also causes hydrostatic distension that allows for easier introduction and advancement of the ureteroscope at the vesicoureteric junction and the rest of the ureter.

The Peditrol is particularly useful if there is a complete or partial ureteric obstruction secondary to a stone. Once the process of stone fragmentation has commenced, the small stone fragments are a nuisance as they get in the way, obscuring vision or interfering with the lithotripsy device. These fragments can be flushed out automatically if the foot pedal is compressed and the ureteroscope is withdrawn at the same time. This reverse slipstream effect happens because there is proximal ureteric obstruction, thus causing the accelerated fluid to return back down the ureter. This flushes the stone fragments downwards and if the ureteroscope is withdrawn at the same time, these fragments fall out of the ureter into the bladder. This obviates the tedious work of removing fragments from the ureter.

It is, however, important to remember that an element of ureteric obstruction is necessary for this to be effective and there is always the risk of proximal stone migration once the stone starts to become smaller with relief of proximal obstruction. This effect would be extremely effective in

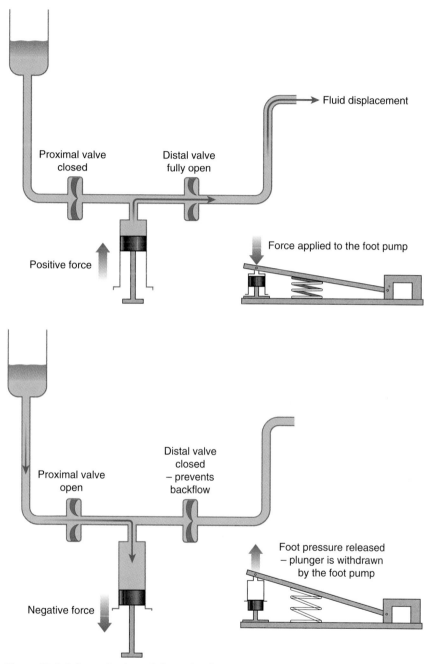

Figure 68.1 Schematic view of the Peditrol.

conjunction with ureteral occlusion devices such as the Accordion (PercSys) or the Backstop (Boston Scientific) as the device can be used to prevent proximal stone migration and the reverse slipstream effect can be used to clear the stone fragments.

The other advantage with the Peditrol is its use in the kidney. Apart from just providing a good flow, the use of the foot pedal makes stones more accessible, especially in the lower pole. After a tipless basket is deployed in the calyx, the accelerated flow from the foot pedal can allow the stone to migrate into the basket, thus enabling extraction. A few pulses with the foot pedal may be necessary before the stone can be snared but it is certainly a useful technique for difficult and inaccessible calyceal stones.

69

Flexible renoscopy and stone fragmentation

Bo Parys

In my practice, if the stone is in the upper pole or I have placed it there for lasertripsy, having previously placed an access sheath up to the pelviureteral junction (PUJ), I advance the scope up to/into the upper pole calyx. Then, under x-ray control, I gently advance the sheath up to or, if it is wide enough, into the neck of the upper pole calyx (Figure 69.1). This ensures that the stone stays trapped during lasertripsy. Small fragments are washed down the access sheath and any fragments that need picking out with a basket are not lost elsewhere in the kidney (Figure 69.2). For this technique to be successful, I always ensure that a hydrophilic sheath is used and kept well lubricated to minimise friction during adjustment of the sheath over the flexible ureterorenoscope.

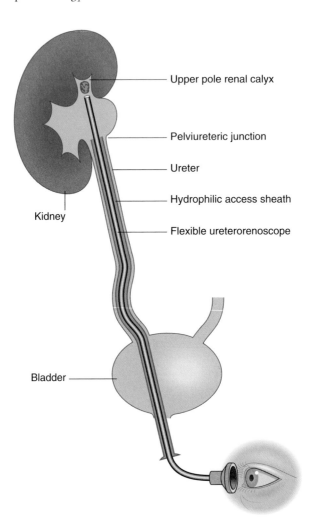

Upper pole renal calyx

Pelviureteric junction

Ureter

Hydrophilic access sheath

Flexible ureterorenoscope

Kidney

Bladder

Figure 69.1 Flexible ureterorenoscope trapping a stone in the upper pole calyx.

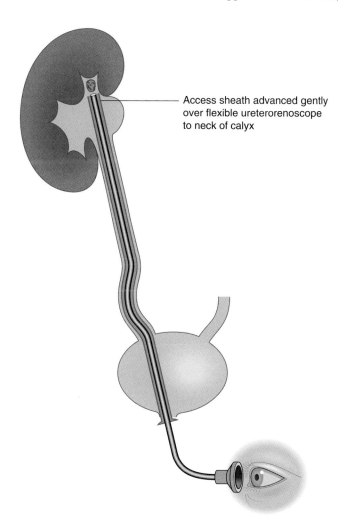

Access sheath advanced gently
over flexible ureterorenoscope
to neck of calyx

Figure 69.2 The access sheath is gently advanced over the flexible ureterorenoscope to the neck of the calyx to minimise stone movement and aid washout of stone fragments.

70

A novel technique to treat large mid or upper ureteric stones

Asif Raza and Muhammad Jamal Khan

Treating large stones (>1 cm maximum diameter) in the mid or upper ureter using a rigid ureteroscope and laser or lithoclast can be difficult. Multiple insertions of the rigid ureteroscope can be time consuming and increase the risk of trauma to the ureter or vesicourethral junction (VUJ) or compromise the view due to bleeding from scope trauma to the ureteric mucosa. This may decrease stone clearance rate and increase the complication rate.

We describe a novel technique which decreases length of procedure and complications and improves stone-free rates. A ureteral access sheath is inserted over a standard guidewire (safety wire) into the kidney. The sheath is placed just proximal to the stone. The stone is fragmented with the use of a flexible ureteroscope and holmium laser. A 28–35 cm access sheath may be used for a midureteric stone or proximal ureteric stone in females and a 45–55 cm sheath for proximal ureteral stones in males.

The diameter of the sheath will depend on whether the patient has a narrow ureter (6–12F sheath). If the patient has been prestented, a 12–14F or 14–16F sheath may be used.

The patient will require a stent at the end of the procedure, which can be removed subsequently.

71

Rigid ureteroscopy

Matthew Bultitude

1 Always check preoperative cultures.
2 Place a safety wire prior to ureteroscopy.
3 To enter the ureteric orifice, it may be necessary to use a second wire through the ureteroscope. It is often necessary to invert the ureteroscope so the two wires separate and open the orifice so the ureteroscope can be passed between the two wires (Figure 71.1).

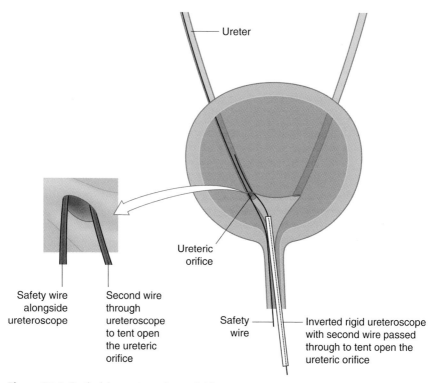

Figure 71.1 Optimising entry using a rigid ureteroscope.

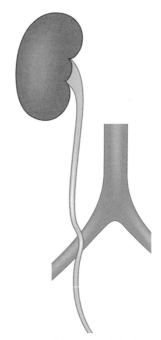

Figure 71.2 The course of the ureter is not a straight line.

4 Remember the course of the ureter. This initially traverses laterally and posterior before curving medially and anterior over the pelvic brim. Finally, it traverses posterior and lateral again up to the renal pelvis. It may be necessary to use a second wire to cross the pelvic brim (Figure 71.2).

5 Keep the irrigation as slow as possible to avoid retropulsion of any stone back into the kidney.

6 There are a number of devices available for preventing retropulsion, e.g. Stone Cone (Boston Scientific), BackStop thermosensitive gel or Accordion stone control device. However, a simple method (depends on channel size of ureteroscope) is to pass a fine-tipped basket (e.g. 2.4 F Segura basket) alongside the stone and open it behind. If the stone rolls back into the basket, the basket can be closed around the stone and the stone further lasered until small enough to remove (Figure 71.3).

7 For awkward upper ureteric stones, consider using a flexible ureteroscope alongside a safety wire. Some surgeons do this routinely for upper ureteric stones.

8 Consider saving time by placing the stent freehand without using the cystoscope. The technique for men and women is different. In the man, deploy the upper curl in the kidney as normal. Then under screening, place the pusher tip at the midpoint of the symphysis pubis. Then withdraw the wire, while holding the pusher in place. The stent should deploy in the

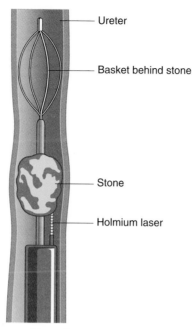

Ureter

Basket behind stone

Stone

Holmium laser

Figure 71.3 Stopping retropulsion of a ureteric stone.

bladder (Figure 71.4). (Note: the pusher must have a radio-opaque marker to use this technique.)

In the woman, the pusher is not even required. After deploying the upper end, push the stent with your index fingernail into the urethra and remove the wire. The lower curl will be deployed into the bladder (Figure 71.4).

Always remember to empty the bladder afterwards!

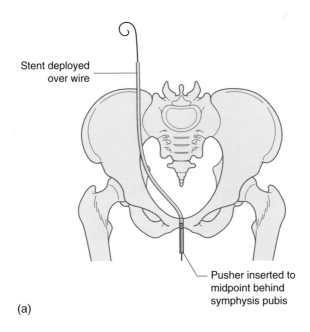

Stent deployed
over wire

Pusher inserted to
midpoint behind
symphysis pubis

(a)

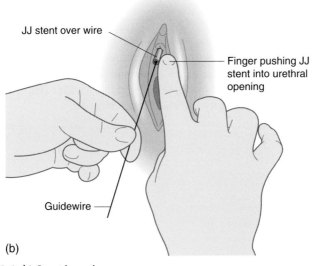

JJ stent over wire

Finger pushing JJ
stent into urethral
opening

Guidewire

(b)

Figure 71.4 (a,b) Stent insertion.

72

The Boston shouldered stent

Bo Parys

I usually use these types of stents for people who have had an endopyelotomy or occasionally other indications. As the stent has a maximum diameter of 14 F, it cannot be passed in the traditional manner through a cystoscope. Given that the stent is too large for cystoscopic passage, I try and pass the stent retrogradely under x-ray control but what often happens is that the guidewire buckles inside the bladder, making stent passage impossible. My trick here, therefore, is to pass the cystoscope sheath over the guidewire and stent and advance it under x-ray control to the ureteric orifice. The rigid structure of the scope prevents the wire from buckling and ensures successful passage of the stent (Figure 72.1).

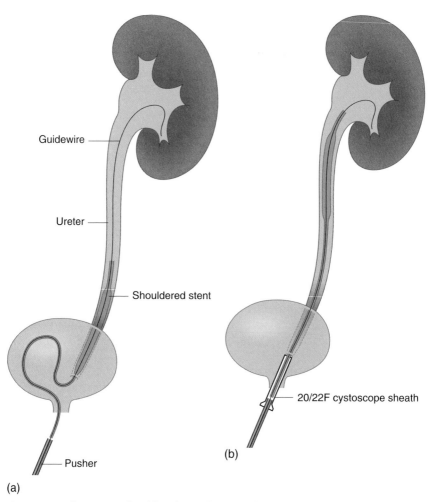

Guidewire

Ureter

Shouldered stent

20/22F cystoscope sheath

(b)

Pusher

(a)

Figure 72.1 The Boston shouldered stent being pushed into position. (a) The guidewire is held straight and then (b) the cystoscope sheath is passed over the wire to act as a more rigid pusher.

73

Ureteroscopy

Nimish Shah

1 During change of JJ stents in patients with chronic conditions necessitating long-term stent placements, firstly always attempt to pass a guidewire alongside the existing stent which acts as a 'road map'. Resist the temptation to pull the existing stent prior to guidewire passage as it may be difficult to identify the ureteric orifice in the presence of marked stent-related inflammation around the ureteric orifice.

2 Always ensure that patients undergoing upper tract endoscopy have preoperative negative voided urine culture to minimise septic complications. Always use antibiotic prophylaxis appropriate to the local guidelines

3 Never attempt upper tract endoscopy or stent placement without the assistance of image intensifier guidance in theatre.

4 Always work with a safety wire in place. If this is not possible immediately, ensure that this is achieved as soon as possible during upper tract endoscopy. This is especially important for ureteric intervention.

5 For primary placement of JJ stents, always perform a retrograde study to establish the exact course of the ureter in order to ensure that the guidewire is appropriately and correctly sited into the renal pelvis, prior to passage of a JJ stent.

6 In order to maximise the durability of your flexible ureteroscope, always consider whether it would be possible to reposition a lower pole stone into an upper (preferably) or midpole calyx prior to laser fragmentation.

7 Always ensure that the flexible ureteroscope is as 'straight' as possible when passing a laser fibre.

8 A 200 μm laser fibre should be the preferred choice when used through a flexible ureteroscope, as this allows greater flexibility and improved irrigation fluid transmission.

9 Always start laser stone fragmentation with a low setting, typically 5 Hz and 0.5 W, only increasing the power if the stone is particularly hard.

10 Use a 'soft hands' approach to upper tract endoscopy; if passage of the ureteroscope during primary ureteroscopy is not possible due to resistance, then avoid using force. A stent placement in such a situation is not

a 'failure', allowing safe return at a later date. Ureteric trauma, on the other hand, with forced passage of a ureteroscope may prove to be a career regret!

11 Try to have 2–4 favoured guidewires and baskets rather than having a very large selection as the latter often proves restrictive, particularly with an unfamiliar theatre team.

12 Try and keep the bladder relatively empty during upper tract endoscopy; an infant feeding tube placed within the bladder during a prolonged case may be helpful. A relatively empty bladder assists with passage of a rigid ureteroscope, especially into the distal ureter.

74

The pinhole scope: part 1

Sunil Kumar and Peter Malone

The ultra thin ureterorenoscope (Richard Wolf GmbH) is a semi-rigid scope with its distal tip measuring only 4.5F and the sheath 6.5F. The lens is 5° with a lateral eyepiece and, more importantly, the instrument channel measures 3.3F, allowing for both diagnostic and therapeutic procedures in the ureter.

This scope can be used for diagnostic ureteric procedures without using a guidewire. It comes into its own if there is a case of failed access with the standard ureteroscope for therapeutic ureteric procedures because of a tight lower ureter. The options at this stage would be to stent the patient and re-do the ureteroscopy in a few weeks' time or do a balloon dilation of the lower ureter. The pinhole scope can circumvent this problem with the additional advantage of having the ability to use most of the disposable instruments necessary to do therapeutic procedures through its 3.3F working channel.

75

Use of the dual-lumen catheter

Oliver Wiseman

A dual-lumen catheter is an invaluable tool for the endourologist. It is used in situations where there is a safety wire *in situ* and the surgeon wishes to perform a retrograde or place a second wire. We use it routinely to place a second wire outside the Amplatz sheath during percutaneous nephrolithotomy (PCNL), prior to dilation of the tract, or to insert a working wire where access to the upper tract is very difficult (e.g. where the patient has an ileal conduit).

The images show a dual-lumen catheter and its use in allowing a flexible ureteroscope to be advanced over a second wire in a patient with an ileal conduit and a renal stone, while still having a safety wire in place (Figures 75.1–75.3).

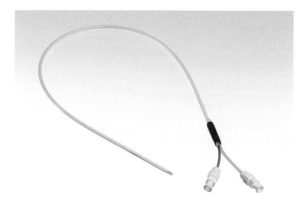

Figure 75.1 A dual-lumen catheter, 10 F diameter, 50 cm length, with two lumens. (With permission from Boston Scientific Corporation.)

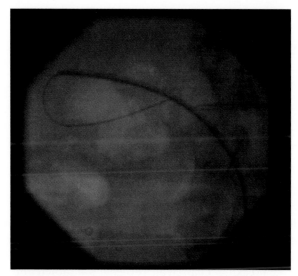

Figure 75.2 A dual-lumen catheter has been advanced retrogradely through the ileal conduit over a safety wire. A second wire is then placed through the dual-lumen catheter.

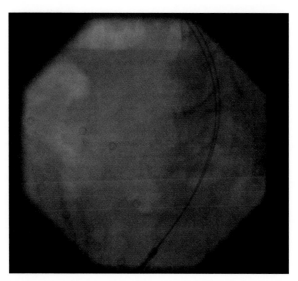

Figure 75.3 The presence of two wires allows the flexible ureteroscope to be advanced over one working wire, leaving a safety wire alongside which facilitates re-entry should, for example, the flexible ureteroscope be withdrawn without placement of a second wire.

76

Flexible ureteroscopy

Stephen Gordon

During flexible ureteroscopy, I had difficulty passing the laser fibre as it seemed to be catching on the inside of the scope. Everything else was passing without difficulty. In order to carry on the case and protect the scope and prevent the fibre breaking, I passed an 18G epidural catheter down the scope with the 200 micron fibre inside it and was able to proceed with reasonable flow still around the catheter. The 200 micron fibre passed down but was tight and at the very tip of the catheter where there are a few holes, the calibre seemed to narrow slightly so the last 1 cm was cut off.

77

Lasering stones

Senthil Nathan

When lasering a stone in the ureter, always hit the side of the stone to slowly chip away the stone. If you hit the centre, either the stone will fly back into the kidney or it will create large fragments and these may fly back into the kidney.

78

Renal pelvic stones

Anthony Blacker

A problem with ureteroscopic management of renal pelvic stones is clearance of the fragments that are generated by the laser. Similar to the effect of the Lithoclast Master, suction can be used on a semi-rigid ureteroscope. Connect suction to the ureteroscope on the opposite side to the irrigation (or use a three-way tap if there is only a single irrigation port). The way to achieve maximum effect is to initially draw the 200–270 micron fibre back until it is just sticking out of the tip of the scope. Even if the laser is not in contact with the stone, start firing, then turn on the suction. Stones and fragments are drawn onto the tip of the laser fibre and resultant dust is automatically aspirated through the scope. The agitation caused by the active laser fibre within the scope prevents dust clogging up the irrigation channel of the ureteroscope. As the renal pelvis is seen collapsing towards the scope tip, stop firing the laser! Normal fragmentation can then be resumed with irrigation, and once the renal pelvis is filled, the cycle can be repeated. This is highly effective at removing all dust and fragments from the renal pelvis, so avoiding the need for a stent even for large renal stones.

79

Difficult urethral stricture encountered at ureteroscopy

James Hall

Passage of the ureteroscope along a freshly urethrotomised urethra is likely to be impossible with all the potential for false passages. I've three times been confronted by very tight, dense, unexpected urethral stricture at planned semi-rigid ureteroscopy for stone and I have each time adopted this technique, which is probably not unique but has worked very well each time.

- Deploy a Sachs urethrotome and Sensor wire through the stricture, allowing safe urethrotomy to be performed.
- With the urethrotome now in the bladder the wire is then passed through the relevant ureteric orifice and to the kidney.
- Place the ureteroscope over this wire.
- Insert a second wire up the ureteroscope to the kidney.
- Remove the ureteroscope, leaving both wires in (safety and working wire), then pass the ureteroscope back in over the working wire to the stone.
- Take the working wire out and perform stone fragmentation.
- Take the ureteroscope out, leaving the safety wire.
- Insert the cystoscope and Albaron bridge over this remaining wire and the JJ stent into the ureter in the usual manner.
- On retraction of the wire from the stent, redeploy a good length of wire into bladder and take the scope out.
- Insert an open-ended 16F catheter over the wire and into the bladder, 10 mL to balloon and take wire out (all done backed up with II screening).
- Perform a trial of catheter in 2–7 days depending on complexity of the urethral stricture.

80

General tips for a simpler and safer ureteroscopy

Sunil Kumar

A preliminary diagnostic cystoscopy is performed and a guide (safety) wire passed up the ureteric orifice under fluoroscopy. A retrograde pyelogram could be performed at this stage if necessary, particularly if there is any problem with free passage of the wire. The cystoscope is now withdrawn, making sure that the safety wire is not dislodged. One of the important steps at this stage is to leave the bladder empty; if the bladder is full, the ureteric orifices are displaced laterally, making access into the lower ureter more difficult. The safety wire needs to be placed in its sheath and clipped away, ensuring that there are no dangling loops that may get caught during the procedure which may lead to its inadvertent dislodgement. Prior to inserting the ureteroscope, it is important to make sure that all attachments are in the right place.

The ureteroscopic image will now need to be white balanced and the focus performed prior to commencing the procedure. It is important to try and not interfere with the focus during the procedure unless it is absolutely essential. The irrigation will also need to be checked to ensure that all the bubbles have been removed as bubbles can really interfere with the ureteroscopy. If the lower ureter or for that matter any part of the ureter is tight, you can always use a second wire to shoe horn the ureter and pass the scope between the two wires.

It is important to remember to keep gentle pressure on the scope when the ureter is tight rather than using active force. Usually the tip of the ureteroscope is narrow and the diameter increases towards the shaft and the proximal end, therefore negotiating the narrow area may not necessarily mean that the rest of the procedure will be easy. The narrow area in the distal ureter may continue to be tight and make it really difficult to pass the ureteroscope. At this stage, it is important to continue to maintain gentle pressure and also to withdraw the scope intermittently to ascertain that the lower ureter is not gripping the scope too tightly as this may rarely lead to intussusception and ureteric avulsion. When the ureteroscope is being withdrawn, you should be able to see the ureteric walls moving away from you, similar to sitting in a train with the landscape moving away; if the landscape is coming with you then you are in trouble.

In patients who have a history of complicated colonic surgery and possibly radiotherapy, it is occasionally difficult to perform a semi-rigid ureteroscopy. I believe the reason for this is that the ureter is fixed within the retroperitoneum as a retrograde usually does not reveal any abnormality. A period of time with a stent *in situ* does not appear to make any difference to a subsequent ureteroscopy. It is therefore necessary in this group of patients to ensure that a flexible ureteroscope is available to perform therapeutic procedures within the ureter.

I cannot stress enough the importance of using contrast and fluoroscopy if there is any difficulty at whatever stage of the procedure just to delineate the anatomy of the ureter and the pelvicalyceal system. Finally, the use of the semi-rigid ureteroscope is underplayed for therapeutic procedures in the renal pelvis or the upper pole. Many of the large renal pelvic and upper pole stones can be dealt with by a semi-rigid scope rather than a flexible ureteroscope. Sometimes even stones in the lower or mid pole calyces can be picked out with the flexible scope and placed in the renal pelvis or upper pole and the semi-rigid scope can then be used to deal with them. I believe that baskets of any shape or form should not be used in the ureter; this has been inculcated in me from my training days in Bristol. A triradiate grasper is the ideal instrument for use in the ureter.

The above tips are not exhaustive but may help in making ureteroscopy easier as we all know how a simple ureteroscopy can suddenly turn out to be not so simple.

81

Flexible ureteroscopy/retrograde study of the right collecting system post cystectomy

Senthil Nathan

At times, a ureteroscopy needs to be done into the right collecting system following a cystectomy. In the Wallace anastomosis the left ureter is in direct line to the ileal conduit. The guidewire frequently goes straight into the left ureter. A simple technique would be to position a guidewire into the left ureter and then to place a Pollack catheter into the left system. Then remove the cystoscope and then insert a guidewire, which will then fly into the right collecting system. A ureteroscope can be passed on this guidewire.

82

Optimising the view for difficult stent insertion

John McLoughlin

It can prove very difficult at times to get a good view inside the bladder with a 30° lens/22 F sheath arrangement. This may be because of debris, a raw bladder wall or even a minor degree of bleeding as may follow a transurethral resection of bladder tumour (TURBT). Typically, you may have a great view whilst resecting a bladder tumour with a resectoscope in use but upon switching to a 22 F sheath, the view deteriorates.

Using a standard optical urethrotomy set (which comes with a small-calibre catheterisation channel, Figure 82.1a) vastly improves your view as the flow characteristics are different from a beaked 22 F sheath. The small channel allows passage of a guidewire – and the wire comes right out where you can see it.

If you can get hold of a long bridge attachment as shown in Figure 82.1, this has an additional larger calibre channel that allows passage of stents as well, which is a really useful attachment. See also Figure 82.2.

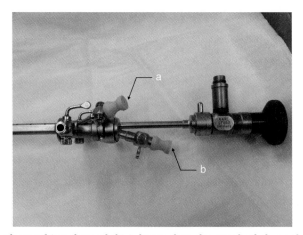

Figure 82.1 The working channel (b) is larger than the standard channel (a) on this extended bridge.

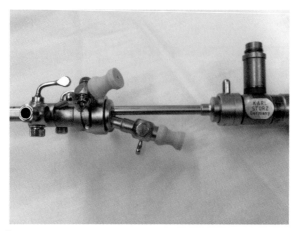

Figure 82.2 Close-up.

If you need to pull the stent, you can simply load a pair of cold cup biopsy forceps and a 30° lens inside the optical working sheath without having to replace the whole sheath.

83

A novel technique for stent exchange over an ileal-ureteric anastomosis

Rob Gray and Hanif Motiwala

We describe a trick for the troublesome change of stent which is placed over an ileal-ureteric anastomosis (Figure 83.1). The stent itself is often encrusted and therefore a guidewire cannot easily be passed through the lumen of the stent once a change is required. Often after removal of the stent, it is not possible to find an opening to insert the guidewire. Our alternative technique utilises an access sheath and is described in easy steps.

1 Using a stent grabber, withdraw the stent from the ileal conduit, leaving the distal end within the ureter.
2 A dual-lumen access sheath or equivalent is rail-roaded over the ureteric stent to the ureteric orifice.
3 A guidewire can then be passed through the lumen of the access sheath (which has cannulated the ureteric orifice) and passed alongside the stent.
4 The stent to be removed can be removed with a guidewire for safety.
5 The stent is then passed over guidewire safely.

Alternatively, the flexible ureteroscope can be passed alongside the stent within the access sheath and the lumen is cannulated with a guidewire, or the stent is removed and the flexible ureteroscope can be inserted directly to the point where it is not possible to push the sheath inside.

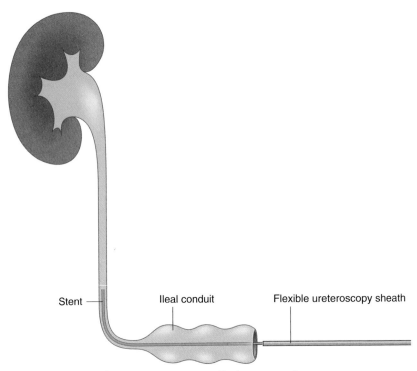

Figure 83.1 Stent exchange over an uretero-ileal anastomosis.

84

Stents

Peter W. Cooke

When inserting stents after ureteroscopy, push the stent pusher through the cystoscope and back feed your safety guidewire through this, rather than putting the wire through the scope directly, getting stuck or having to take the scope apart.

85

Placing a stent in a female patient without having to reload the cystoscope or performing a stent change in a female patient with a flexible cystoscope only

Gerald Rix

The patient is placed in the usual lithotomy position. The stent is then grasped and removed until it just protrudes from the urethra. A new guidewire can be threaded down it. The stent is then removed over the guidewire. A new stent is then threaded over the guidewire and pushed with the finger until the finger is pushing quite firmly against the external urethral meatus. The image intensifier is used as normal to check the upper coil and then the guidewire is withdrawn whilst preventing the stent from slipping back out by maintaining pressure on the external urethral meatus. As the guidewire comes out of the bottom coil, this will usually spring up the urethra and assume its normal position in the bladder. The position can be checked with a quick flash of the image intensifier. If the lower coil still remains within the urethra, it is a relatively simple matter to just pass the rigid scope with the blind obturator, if doing this under general anaesthetic, or alternatively with the flexible cystoscope if doing this under local, in order to push the coil into the correct position on the bladder.

This saves having to thread the guidewire through the cystoscope in order to place the stent under direct vision. Clearly, this method only works in female patients.

86

Paired JJ stents for retroperitoneal fibrosis

John McLoughlin

Patients with retroperitoneal fibrosis are often frail, present with renal impairment and end up having one or more nephrostomies inserted. These can usually be internalised by antegrade stents placed by the radiologist so as to allow subsequent removal of nephrostomy.

However, on occasion, the JJ stent will not drain as well as a nephrostomy as it is compressed externally. There are specific triradiate stents that can be ordered for this situation but as a simple trick, a second stent in the same ureter can also be used as it produces a gap between the contours of stents that allows urine to percolate (Figure 86.1, *arrows*).

My tips to optimise the chance of getting a second stent into what is effectively a tight ureter are:

- insert *both* wires at the beginning, then and only then rail-road the stents directly in under x-ray guidance into correct position
- leave the string on the stent and guidewire *in situ* until you are happy with the position of both stents as the first may slip up the ureter as the second is rail-roaded, requiring adjustment of its position
- you may need to use a standard 6 and a smaller 4.8 stent together if two larger stents will not pass.

In my experience, this works best for female patients.

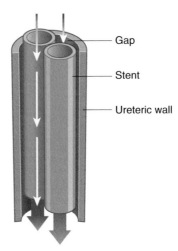

Figure 86.1 Paired bilateral JJ stents.

87

Four tips relating to ureteric stenting

Sunil Kumar

1 Once a decision has been made about stenting the patient, it is important to have an idea of the length and diameter of the stent that you are going to use. Adult stents can vary in length from 24 to 30 cm and there are also multi-length stents that can go up to 32 cm. On an average patient, a 26 cm stent is ideal; in shorter patients a 24 cm stent is adequate. I personally discourage the use of the multi-length stent as occasionally you can end up with multiple coils in the renal pelvis that can cause all sorts of problems, such as failure to uncoil or even knotting of the stent during extraction. We have all experienced encrustation of the stent within the bladder and unfortunately the same thing can also happen in the renal pelvis. In addition, there has been some recent evidence to suggest that the longer the length of the stent in the bladder, the more symptomatic it is for the patient. It is important to be aware that there is a 4.8/4.7F stent that can be used for narrow strictures or to bypass stones that may not allow a standard 6F stent.

2 We have all encountered the stent that either does not come out after a few tugs with reasonable force or gets stuck in the ureter. If there is a large stone at the top end of the stent then it is highly likely that a percutaneous extraction would be required. My advice now would be to put an artery clip if part of the stent is outside the urethra to prevent it from slipping back inside again. A ureteroscopy is now essential and this has to be performed alongside the stent up the ureter, dealing with any encrustation along the way with the holmium laser. The artery clip will help to keep the stent from slipping back again and also helps with countertraction which may release the stent. Once again, the pinhole scope is extremely useful for this procedure. The ureteroscope can be passed all the way to the kidney if required.

3 A simple tip to insert a stent after the ureteroscope is removed with the safety wire in place is to pass the pusher up the bridge of the cystoscope and backload the safety wire through the lumen of the pusher. The pusher can then be removed and the cystoscope introduced over the guidewire. Once in the bladder, the stenting can proceed as usual. An open-ended ureteric catheter can be used for this purpose.

4 I recommend that the anatomy of the pelvicalyceal system is always delineated prior to stenting; in other words, a retrograde should always be performed prior to stent insertion so that the stent can be placed precisely. To this end, I also advise that the string attached to the stent is used for this purpose. The string attached to the end of the stent can be utilised for various purposes. It helps to position or reposition the stent precisely. If the guidewire slips or falls out during stent insertion, the string is useful to pull the stent out without needing to revert to the biopsy forceps. Once the stent is positioned, the string is cut and the assistant pulls the string out whilst the surgeon maintains countertraction on the pusher. If this is not done, the stent can be dislodged. Once the string is removed, the guidewire and the pusher can be extracted.

88

Insertion of JJ stent

Senthil Nathan

When a JJ stent is being inserted, after positioning a guidewire frequently a portion of the stent goes into the ureter and then stops. Even with pressure and countertraction, the stent will not advance forward and the reason for this is that when there is laxity or resistance, the stent tends to migrate within the cystoscope sheath laterally. One trick is to undo the sheath slightly and then advance the stent and then lock the bridge back onto the telescope. This will straighten the guidewire and stent and then it will advance smoothly.

89

Basketing of stones

Senthil Nathan

When basketing small stones, the basket should be kept very close to the ureteroscope. If the basket is kept away from the ureteroscope then it will sag onto the ureteric mucosa and when the basket is closed, it will pull the mucosa and injure it. A simpler technique would be to just pull the basket into the ureteroscope so it closes by its retraction rather than using the handle.

90

Backloading guidewires

David Hendry

This tip was standard practice in Ayr and I think may have been written up some years ago by Abu Rani who described backloading a guidewire onto a cystoscope for stent changes, etc. This is really very simple, in that a ureteric catheter, or the pusher that comes with the stent, is placed forwards through the cystoscope, allowing the guidewire to be backloaded through the pusher or ureteric catheter, which can then be removed and the guidewire is then positioned perfectly through the scope.

91

Insertion of a guidewire into the ureter

Senthil Nathan

Frequently, the guidewire skids off the ureter when attempting to insert it. The trick would be to turn the scope entirely upside down so that you are looking directly on to the ureteric orifice and the guidewire will go perpendicular to the opening of the ureteric orifice.

92

A solution for stent-related bladder symptoms

Paul Halliday

Many patients suffer bladder pain or irritability in relation to the presence of a ureteric stent and this can be difficult to manage in patients who require a stent long term. Provided that there is no obstruction of the distal ureter, this problem can be overcome by removing the lower coil together with perhaps 2.3 cm of the bottom end of the stent and attaching a loop of 2/0 non-absorbable suture material approximately 10 cm in circumference. The stent should be divided 5 mm below one of the side holes and the suture passed through the side hole before trying to complete the loop. This allows easy removal of the stent without any folding or buckling of the bottom end. The stent can then be placed in the normal way, leaving only a loop of suture material protruding 2.3 cm into the bladder.

See Figure 92.1.

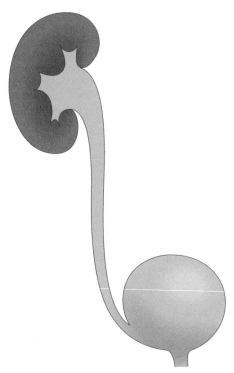

Figure 92.1 Stent stays out of the bladder. The guidewire passes into the bladder and allows the stent to be easily grabbed.

PART 4
Lower Urinary Tract

Top Tips in Urology, Second Edition. Edited by John McLoughlin, Neil Burgess, Hanif Motiwala, Mark J. Speakman, Andrew Doble and John D. Kelly.
© 2013 John Wiley & Sons, Ltd. Published 2013 by John Wiley & Sons, Ltd.

93

Holmium laser enucleation of the prostate: laser technique

Tev Aho

When making the 5 and 7o'clock bladder neck incisions (BNIs):
- at the proximal end, cut vertically down through the lip of the bladder neck until you can look straight across the trigone (Figure 93.1)
- at the distal end, position the fibre tip on the floor at the midpoint of the veru and incise horizontally to enter the tissue plane under the apex of the lateral lobe. This is the easiest place to get into the enucleation plane (Figure 93.2).

When enucleating the median lobe:
- use the beak of the scope to nudge under the bottom edge of the lobe, holding it up under tension to laser against and peel up (Figure 93.3)
- keep freeing up the lateral corners of the lobe whilst advancing it (Figure 93.4)
- sit at the bladder neck edge with the fibre tip and incise horizontally left and right when detaching. Do not laser up onto the trigone.

When enucleating the lateral lobes:
- begin by placing the fibre tip alongside the veru at its midpoint and rotating the instrument up and around as far as possible towards 12o'clock (see Figure 93.2)
- with the instrument rotated through 180° and the fibre tip at a level just proximal to the veru, laser vertically up and then across to mark the distal extent of the 12o'clock BNI and enter the plane anterior to the apex (Figure 93.5a,b)
- complete the 12o'clock BNI in a retrograde direction (Figure 93.5b)
- detach the apex from the external sphincter as early as possible. If unsure what is still holding the apex in place, pull back to the bulbar urethra to identify any mucosal bridges still attached to the apex (Figure 93.6). Rotational movements with the scope here often aid in identifying the sides of a mucosal bridge.

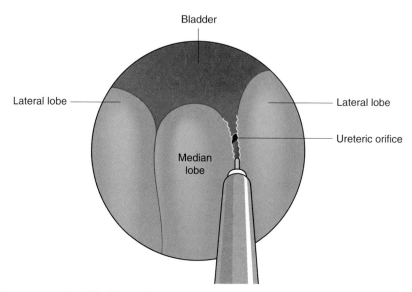

Figure 93.1 Initial bladder neck incision, repeated bilaterally.

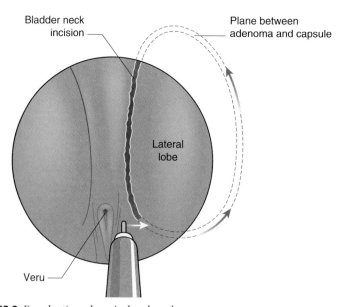

Figure 93.2 Enucleation plane is developed.

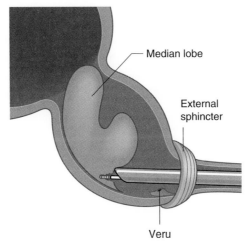

Figure 93.3 The approach to the median lobe.

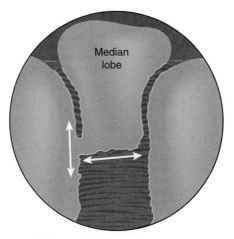

Figure 93.4 Detachment of the median lobe.

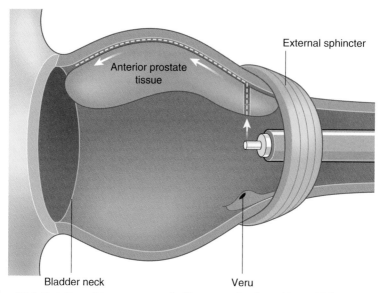

Figure 93.5 Rotation of instrument to facilitate enucleation of lateral lobes.

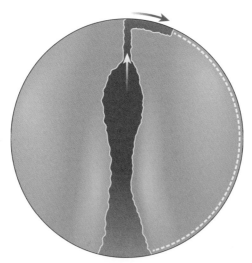

Figure 93.6 Detachment of mucosal bridge. Rotation of scope can help identify any remaining tissue attachments.

94

Holmium laser enucleation of the prostate: safe morcellation

Tev Aho

- Ensure excellent haemostasis at the completion of the laser phase.
- Attach two fluid giving sets to the nephroscope and turn any outflow taps off. This helps maintain a fully distended bladder.
- Approach prostate tissue from underneath. Suck and activate the blades momentarily to attach prostate tissue to the anterior aspect of the morcellator blades over the window.
- Drop hands down to raise the tip of the blades and attached prostate up into the middle of the bladder, then begin morcellation.
- Stop morcellation if prostate tissue is not completely covering the window on the blades.
- If small prostate pieces bounce off the blades, slow the blade speed to help keep them attached.
- To avoid 'chasing' small prostate pieces around, stop inflow briefly and wait for them to settle on the bladder base. Then suction them onto blades and recommence irrigation before reactivating the blades.
- Use graspers, a cold loop or an Ellick to remove very small pieces.

95

Holmium cystolitholapaxy

Sunil Kumar

Endoscopic removal of bladder stones can be difficult, especially if they are large, hard, smooth and multiple. Hence the preferred method of treating these stones is usually an open cystolithotomy. This does have some implications in terms of postoperative recovery and the need for an indwelling catheter, at least for a few days.

The 100 watt holmium laser cuts through bladder stones like a knife through butter and all bladder stones, regardless of size and number, can be fragmented. The power can be modified depending upon the hardness of the stone but if performed appropriately, the procedure will reduce the stone to dust or small fragments that can be washed out easily. It is better performed with a continuous flow scope with a special fibre channel. It can also be used with a standard resectoscope or even a cystoscope with the 500 micron laser fibre inserted through a ureteric catheter. The ureteric catheter helps to keep the laser fibre stable. If there are multiple large stones, procedure time could be long and if required a holmium laser enucleation of the prostate could be performed at the same time. A catheter may be left in overnight if required.

96

Transurethral resection of prostate 1

Nikesh Thiruchelvam

At the end of a transurethral resection of prostate (TURP) procedure, I inflate the three-way catheter to the approximate size of the cavity (there is a French paper showing that, wherever you think you have put the balloon, by filling with contrast, it always ends up sitting in the prostatic cavity rather than at the bladder neck). If you have a large cavity, you can fill the balloon to more than 100 mL if needed. I then pull on the catheter to create traction (regardless of the colour of the irrigation) and then wait while the theatre team around me are removing all the chips, putting the legs down and getting ready to transfer the patient. I then stop my traction when the patient has transferred to the bed. This has usually resulted in 5 min of excellent traction and clear urine!

97

Transurethral resection of prostate 2

Peter W. Cooke

After transurethral resection of prostate (TURP), consistent catheter traction is best achieved by tightly tying an opened out blue gauze swab around the catheter and sliding it right up to the urethral meatus, thus pulling the catheter down. Even if the patient moves, it keeps the traction on.

98

Transurethral vaporisation of the prostate

Senthil Nathan

When vaporising the prostate using a rollerball or a VaporTrode, charring frequently occurs on the rollerball when using cutting current. To clear the debris from the rollerball, press the quiet button and run it along the prostate. This will clear all charred debris.

99

Use of catheter introducer

Derek Fawcett

Increasing the rigidity of the urethral catheter by means of a metal introducer is a required skill of urological practice when simple insertion has failed, often after several attempts ending up with blood on the catheter tip, indicating a false passage.

A catheter introducer is a dangerous weapon, with the potential to make false passages worse. Use carefully.

Tips

- *The patient is often distressed*: give analgesia.
- *The urethra is a straight midline structure*: straighten the patient, pelvis and legs in the bed.
- *All false new passages are POSTERIOR*: LIFT and introduce, don't push.

100

An alternative way to pass a urethral catheter post transurethral resection of prostate

Ben Ayres and Gary Das

While performing transurethral resection of prostate (TURP), there is a risk of undermining the bladder neck when passing a three-way irrigating catheter at the end of the procedure. To reduce this risk, introducers are used to curve the catheter, allowing it to follow the anatomy of the urethra more closely. However, sometimes this curve remains too oblique, resulting in difficult urethral catheterisation and risking the formation of a false passage.

An alternative technique which the senior author has used successfully on many occasions is to use a fine Clutton sound dilator as an introducer as this gives the tip of the catheter a more acute curve, allowing it to negotiate the bulbar urethra and resected bladder neck more easily. This technique involves inserting the tip of a 6/10 or 8/12 gauge Clutton sound dilator into the eye at the end of the catheter in a similar manner to inserting a Maryfield introducer.

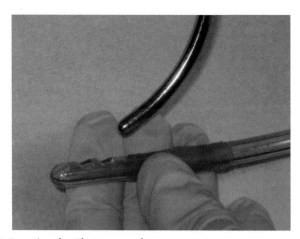

Figure 100.1 Inserting the Clutton sound.

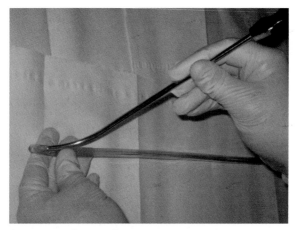

Figure 100.2 Clutton sound inserted into eye of catheter.

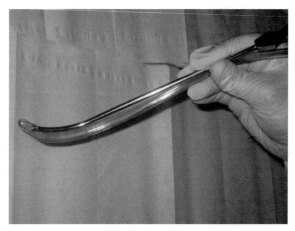

Figure 100.3 View of set-up.

The remainder of the catheter is held adjacent to the shaft of the dilator. After adequate lubrication, the dilator and catheter are gently passed into the urethra just as one would perform a urethral dilation. Once the bulbar urethra, resected prostatic cavity and bladder neck are passed and the combined dilator and catheter are inside the bladder, the Clutton sound can be gently withdrawn whilst the catheter remains in the bladder and the catheter balloon can then be inflated.

See Figures 100.1–100.3.

101

The 17F integral cystoscope

Graham Sole

The 17F integral cystoscope was designed by Ron Miller in the early 1980s and manufactured by GU (Figure 101.1). I have used it for over 20 years and find it invaluable.

The 30° lens and it's 17F instrument channel are integrated. The tip is smooth and bevelled for gentle introduction through the meatus (Figure 101.2).

Advantages

- The small calibre reduces postoperative discomfort.
- A diathermy electrode or ureteric catheter is held firmly and appears exactly in the centre of view.
- When using a ureteric catheter to push a stone, this enables firm pressure to be applied without the catheter coiling in the bladder.
- Biopsy and low-power diathermy can be precisely delivered in the urethra.
- Difficult strictures can be dilated by passing a guidewire and rail-roading the scope itself through the stricture or alternatively a fine (5F), long, Porges filiform bougie can be passed through the stricture and graduated follow-on dilators attached once the scope has been removed over the filiform.

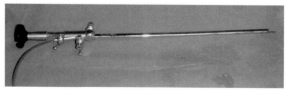

Figure 101.1 The integrated cystoscope.

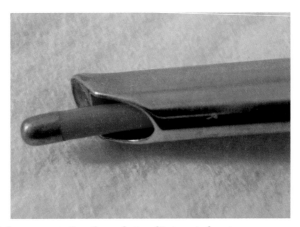

Figure 101.2 Instrumentation through tip of integrated cystoscope.

Disadvantages

- Slow to fill and empty bladder.
- Narrow-angle lens requires inspection of the anterior wall/bladder neck before the bladder becomes too full.

The original model is no longer available but the Storz 27035 BA is similar although the instrument channel is smaller and offset which prevents the use of straight metal instruments. A size 6F stent can be inserted with this instrument.

When my time comes to be cystoscoped, I hope my urologist will consider using this small-calibre, patient-friendly scope!

102

Non-irrigating resectoscope

Graham Sole

One of the main morbidities of transurethral resection of the prostate (TURP) is postoperative stricturing. Otis urethrotomy has been shown to reduce this complication but before doing this, consider using a smaller instrument.

The inner sheath of a Storz 26F irrigating resectoscope is 24F and works perfectly well as long as you are willing to patiently empty the bladder when full!

103

Urethral strictures

Anthony Blacker

When a tight urethral stricture is found at flexible cystoscopy, rather than booking a general anaesthetic (GA) urethrotomy, pass a Sensor guidewire through the working channel of the scope and through the stricture under direct vision. The stricture can then be dilated up to 21F using a balloon dilator over the guidewire. Some balloons can be passed through the scope. For others, the scope needs to be removed from the wire for the balloon to pass over the guidewire, and the scope can be passed alongside to observe the dilation. I do not normally leave a catheter after this procedure. It is well tolerated without anaesthesia for bulbar strictures but painful for meatal strictures, so my preference for those is to use lidocaine injection around the meatus using an insulin syringe.

104

Assessment of paediatric urethral strictures

Amjad Mumtaz Peracha

Paediatric cystoscopies are generally recommended to assess the site, severity and extent of urethral strictures prior to optical urethrotomy but as paediatric cystoscopes are not generally available in most adult urology units, I tend to use the short ureteroscope which has proven very useful and popular in our department. It not only helps to assess the stricture itself but also allows one to leave a guidewire in the bladder prior to optical urethrotomy. The guidewire can also be used to aid insertion of an open-tipped urethral catheter after the procedure, avoiding the need to use a split sheath with the optical urethrotome, which makes it quite bulky.

The pinhole scope: part 2

Sunil Kumar and Peter Malone

The ultra thin ureterorenoscope (Richard Wolf GmbH) is a semi-rigid scope with its distal tip measuring only 4.5F and the sheath is 6.5F. The lens is 5° with a lateral eyepiece and more importantly, the instrument channel measures 3.3F.

Internal optical urethrotomy should be a simple operation. The urethral stricture, usually in the bulb, is cut internally with a cold blade under direct vision usually using a Sachse urethrotome. Nevertheless, it is an operation that from time to time goes wrong, particularly with long dense strictures, when the surgeon cuts outside the urethra and can't find the lumen to proceed. Not infrequently, a flap develops and the operation has to be abandoned, leaving the patient to the pain of urinary retention with the only rescue by suprapubic catheter.

In order to minimise this risk, the wise surgeon passes a guidewire or fine catheter through the stricture into the bladder so that there is always a guide to follow if the surgeon gets lost. The problem arises if the wire will not pass or if it does not pass all the way. As a registrar, I've cursed more than once as the guidewire flipped out of the urethra just at the most crucial time and over the course of my years as a consultant, I've seen many others make the same mistake.

The reason it hasn't happened to me for many a year is that I now make absolutely certain that the guidewire is well curled up in the bladder before I start the urethrotomy. The fine tip of the pinhole ureteroscope can get through nearly all strictures and on the rare occasions that it does not, the working channel is big enough to accept a guidewire so it can be rail-roaded as a gentle dilator under vision. To get reasonable vision, it is necessary to pressurise the irrigant bag or the flow is too poor through the fine working channel. The guidewire should be passed as far as possible and when the entrance to the stricture has been gently dilated, it is usually easy to see the way forward to inch the wire further until the stricture has been negotiated. Once in the bladder, the guidewire can be curled several times around, making it virtually impossible to accidentally dislodge before removing the pinhole scope over it. An additional benefit is that the gentle dilation of the stricture allows slightly better flow of irrigant during the urethrotomy, ensuring good vision.

It can also act as a useful adjunct to urethrography when assessing the length of a stricture prior to urethroplasty. Its additional uses are for ureteric procedures in children. This scope is certainly a valuable addition to a urologist's armamentarium.

How to remove air bubbles in the dome of the bladder

David Hendry

I learned this tip from Colin Bunce. Air bubbles in the dome of the bladder are a common problem and it is a common site of recurrence. The tip he gives is that when using an irrigating resectoscope, you swap over the ingoing irrigation onto the outlet of the scope, put the beak of the scope up in amongst the air bubbles and open the tap which was the inlet tap and the air is all removed. This then gives perfect vision of the dome of the bladder to allow biopsy, resection and diathermy of the recurrences.

107

Resecting multiple bladder tumours

Senthil Nathan

When there are multiple lesions in the bladder, one must resect the lesions starting from the base. If you remember emptying a dishwasher, it will help you to resect the lesions one by one from the base on to the dome of the bladder. This is to avoid blood dropping from the dome of the bladder.

108

Primary transurethral resection of bladder tumour

Aasem Chaudry

During primary transurethral resection of bladder tumour (TURBT), always biopsy the edge separately. Tumour edge biopsy in all primary TURBTs is recommended in the European Association of Urology (EAU) guidelines but is not widely practised in the UK. Our experience of 55 cases indicates that unexpected histopathology is seen in 30% of cases and alters the management in up to 20% of cases with superficial disease.

Technique: TURBT is completed as standard. After completion of the procedure, a cold cup biopsy forceps is used to take a biopsy of the edge of the resection site.

109

Trawling for flat superficial bladder tumour

John McLoughlin

I am always surprised to see trainees struggling with flat superficial transitional cell carcinoma (TCC) of the bladder because they are unaware of this technique. I first saw this described in the first edition of *Top Tips* 20 years ago by David Arkell from Dudley and have used it ever since. The technique here is slightly modified.

The problem is that for flat widespread superficial TCC, there is a tendency to dig holes in some areas and leave other areas under-resected – the 'hills and valley' technique. This method allows you to skim across under the tumour at a predetermined depth.

First, make sure the current in the cutting diathermy is engaged a fraction of a second before the loop touches tissue and not just after. Otherwise you will instinctively dig to try make the loop cut (it is a little like having to apply a lot of force to make your first skin incision because the knife is blunt).

Next, gently push the loop down vertically through the bladder wall with the current on but without bringing the loop inwards until you reach your desired depth (Figure 109.1).

Start your resection by slowly pulling the resectoscope with the loop fully open back along the bladder wall at a depth just deeper than the tumour for the length of the tumour (trawling) (Figure 109.1a). This is best done by sitting slightly further back from the tumour than usual and by using both hands to manipulate the resectoscope so that the usual fulcrum effect is reduced (Figure 109.1b). As you reach the margin of the tumour then finally bring in the loop towards the beak to cut free the tissue as the loop engages the beak (Figure 109.1c). If you need to go deeper, just repeat.

Start on one side (left or right) and work towards the centre of the tumour. Then move to the other side and repeat.

For big bushy tumours I resect the tip as for a transurethal resection of prostate (TURP) then resect the base as described above.

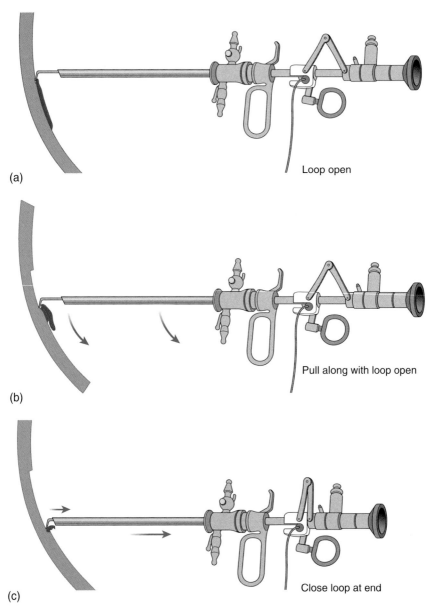

(a)

Loop open

(b)

Pull along with loop open

(c)

Close loop at end

Figure 109.1 (a–c) Trawling for bladder tumour. Keep the loop open and stand back! Only close the loop at the very end.

110

Resecting bladder tumours

Richard Bell

Angling the loop to 45° and minimally filling the bladder whilst resecting posterior wall bladder tumours allows for a safe resection.

111

Never use an Ellick in a clot retention

Simon Bott

There is a temptation to use the Ellick evacuator to remove a clot in patients with clot retention. However, there is a risk that this will cause bladder rupture in an already distended bladder. I therefore suggest inserting a resectoscope sheath, applying the connector and rubber tubing that attaches to an Ellick and then an empty bladder syringe. Try aspirating via the bladder syringe to remove the clot. Do not instil any more fluid. If this fails then I find using a resectoscope without any electricity to 'resect' the clot piecemeal is an effective and safe way of dealing with the problem.

112

Displaced suprapubic catheter

Dan Wilby and Matt Hayes

To avoid the morbidity associated with the formal resiting of a suprapubic catheter that has been removed with unsuccessful attempts to replace, the apparently 'closed' suprapubic tract can often be canalised with a standard guidewire and safely dilated using the plastic dilators provided in a Seldinger type kit. As an alternative, use sequential hollow urethral dilators (Cook).

PART 5
Andrology

Top Tips in Urology, Second Edition. Edited by John McLoughlin, Neil Burgess,
Hanif Motiwala, Mark J. Speakman, Andrew Doble and John D. Kelly.
© 2013 John Wiley & Sons, Ltd. Published 2013 by John Wiley & Sons, Ltd.

113

Glans 'droop' following the insertion of a penile prosthesis

Asif Muneer, Suks Minhas and Alex Kirkham

Patients may develop a glans droop, also known as an 'SST deformity', following the insertion of a penile prosthesis, be it a malleable or an inflatable implant. The deformity can be the result of the tips of the implant being too short or secondary to the anatomical variation in the glans. If the tips of the prosthesis are in the correct position then the deformity can be corrected by performing a glanspexy. Short implants require dilation of the corpora and upsizing. Where there is difficulty in deciding on the underlying cause, penile magnetic resonance imaging (MRI) can be performed to demonstrate the position of the implant although a simpler method would be to perform an ultrasound scan of the glans in order to assess whether the tips are too short.

Figure 113.1 illustrates the appearance of the glans and corpora with the implant inflated postoperatively. Gentle pressure on the glans (Figure 113.2)

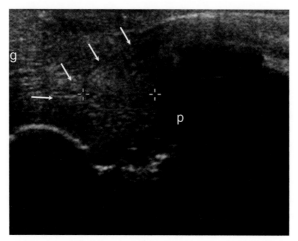

Figure 113.1 Longitudinal ultrasound of the penis demonstrating the tip of the prosthesis relative to the tunica. Arrows mark the tunica around the corpus cavernosum. p, prosthesis; g, glans.

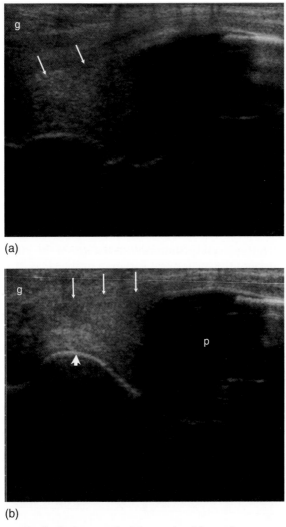

(a)

(b)

Figure 113.2 Longitudinal ultrasound of the penis with gentle pressure on the glans penis. Pressure on the glans (g) from a finger (*arrowhead*) moves the tip of the corpus and glans (b) compared to at rest (a), even with the prosthesis (p) fully inflated.

demonstrates that the tips are approximately 1 cm too short. In this particular case, the rear tips were exchanged for some which were 1 cm longer following redilation of the corpora and the glans droop subsequently resolved.

114

The key to a successful epididymectomy: the bungee manoeuvre

John McLoughlin

Careful selection is essential. My own feeling is that unless you have had a vasectomy, you shouldn't be having an epididymectomy for pain as the success is much lower. The ideal selection is a patient who has a tender epididymis starting at the time of vasectomy; typically it is unilateral. If patients have bilateral pain I would do one side only and see if it worked before progressing to the other after a period of follow-up.

Initial dissection involves taking the epididymis off the side wall of the testis. I create a series of windows so that the epididymis is bow-stringed up and keep as close as humanly possible to the epididymis using clips and no diathermy. I then proceed proximally as far along the vas as the vasectomy site, taking the vasectomy site with the specimen. Distally I take it right to the rete testis; it is important not to leave even a smidgen of tissue there as this will cause a tender bobble on the testicle for some time after. The procedure is much more difficult if you start at one end and work along to the other end. It is much better to get both ends (head and vas site) dissected off and work inwards from both directions.

When you are at a stage where you have two ends that are detached, you are usually left with an area that looks very non-anatomical and adjacent to the vasculature. Herein lays the real trick. What I then do is to pull one end through to the other side (Figure 114.1) and then use both ends as traction to create a bridge of tissue that can be safely clipped. This was nick-named the 'bungee manoeuvre' years ago by one of our trainees – when you try it you will see why.

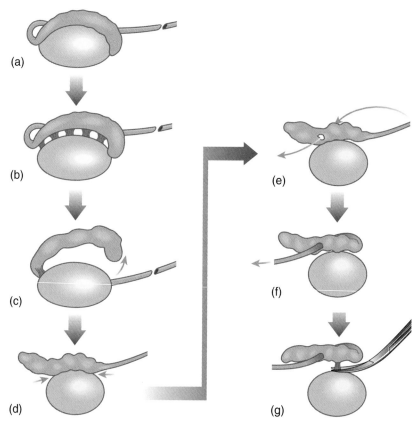

Figure 114.1 (a–g) The bungee manoeuvre. Once both ends are mobilised, pull the vas through the portion of the epididymis that lies nearest to the vasculature to minimise risk of injury.

115

Haemostasis for Nesbit's procedure

Suks Minhas

The Nesbit's procedure for Peyronie's is a common procedure performed by most urologists. However, on occasion all surgeons can run into difficulties, especially when trying to achieve haemostasis during and after the operation. If a large haematoma develops postsurgically then always evacuate this as subsequently patients will develop contracture of the penis and in some instances chronic pain which can be quite debilitating.

I always perform surgery through a circumferential incision, and in most cases will circumcise the patient. With all circumcisions there is a tendency to bleed, therefore ensure that you have sutured the frenular area as if you just use diathermy alone in these cases then subsequently on performing artificial erection, bleeding can be triggered from these diathermied areas by the saline infusion. I tend to reconstruct the frenular area with Vicryl.

When degloving the penis, ensure that you are in between the plane of the dartos and Buck's fascia. If you are not in this plane you will often cause bleeding. Ensure that you use a mixture of sharp and blunt dissection to deglove the penis down. Often there will be vessels that are perforated between the two layers. I always ligate these. Once the penis is degloved, always ensure that you evert the dartos upwards, so that you can inspect around to ensure that there are no bleeding vessels that need to be ligated. Often in re-do surgery, Buck's fascia will be very adherent to the dartos muscle itself and it can be quite difficult to stop the bleeding vessels. The area that particularly bleeds is that between the urethra and the dartos, so ensure that haemostasis is maintained here as often there is a paraurethral vessel that runs close by between the dartos and the spongiosum of the ure-thra. When incising the Buck's fascia, ensure that you tie large vessels, as often if you just diathermy these they will bleed during the artificial erection process, which can be a nuisance.

Often the urethra will need to be partially or totally mobilised for most curvatures, and therefore ensure that you are in the right plane from the start. Small tears of the urethral spongiosum can bleed quite a lot. Always mobilise the urethra with a catheter to try and prevent small lacerations. In fact, I perform all Nesbit's with the patient catheterised. Occasionally, an open sinus will bleed from the urethra and in these cases the urethra can be superficially oversown with a 5/0 Vicryl suture.

After performing the Nesbit's plication, which I perform with PDS sutures, there is often quite profuse bleeding from the suture sites or in between. In these cases I often use a Vicryl 3/0 suture to oversew the area at the bleeding points.

The key to haemostasis in the Nesbit's procedure, and avoiding a large haematoma, is to ensure that the Buck's fascia is sutured in continuity on each side. This layer acts as a haemostatic barrier that often prevents spread of haematoma into the dartos layer. I suture this with a 3/0 Vicryl stitch. Occasionally (particularly on a re-do procedure), the dartos layer will fragment and tear on suturing and in these cases if it does tear then tie the Vicryl stitch at that point, and then start with another suture to prevent excessive tension in the area which may cause further tearing.

At the end of the procedure make sure the penis is flaccid as partially erect penises can clearly bleed further.

If you still find that the area is bleeding or oozing, then a light compression dressing can be used in these circumstances, but ensure that the patient is catheterised and you do not use the pressure dressing unless you have circumcised the patient. If the patient is not circumcised then the pressure dressing can cause distal necrosis of the skin, distal to the circumferential incision – a complication which I have seen.

116

Nesbit's procedure

John McLoughlin

None of these tips is original to myself bar the lock-out valve tip, but all have some merit.

Use an Allis forceps to pinch the corpora on the side away from the Peyronie's plaque. Adjust the jaws to alter the volume of tissues grabbed and in doing so, the degree of correction achieved. After about 30 sec, this leaves a mark that allows you to mark out where your incision and/or sutures are to be placed (Figure 116.1).

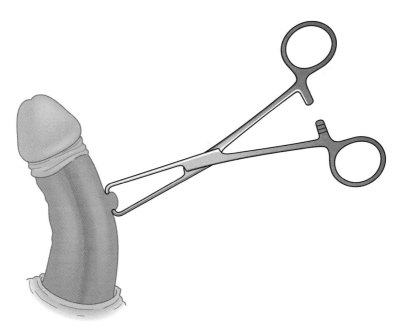

Figure 116.1 Allis forceps used to grasp the exposed corporal body.

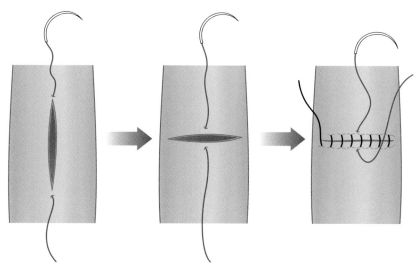

Figure 116.2 Corporotomy apical sutures.

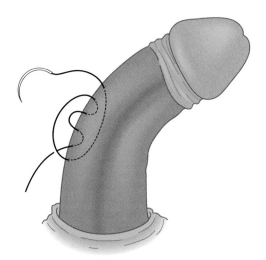

Figure 116.3 'Correction and tension-relieving' stitch.

Should you perform a corporal incision and a plasty type correction, try inserting a (PDS) suture at the apex of each end of the incision in order to mark out the half-way point so that you achieve maximum correction with your sutures. Otherwise you can get a 'collapsed' square which doesn't work as well (Figure 116.2).

I also like a 'correction and tension-relieving' stitch to correct curvatures in younger patients. The first passes of the suture simply plicate the corpora.

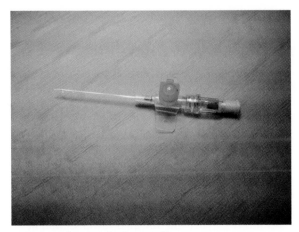

Figure 116.4 Lock-out valve attached to Venflon.

After the suture exits the corporal body, the suture is pulled tight to produce the correction. The suture is then passed back deeper through the corporal bodies and used to tie over the plication to relieve tension and also to reduce the chances of the suture cutting out (Figure 116.3).

I use a lock-out valve (obtainable from the anaesthetist) to stop the saline used to reproduce an intraoperative erection bleeding back and deflating the erection prematurely (Figure 116.4).

117

Tension-free vasectomy reversal

Asif Muneer

As with all anastomotic surgery, the finished result should be tension free in order to avoid failure or restenosis. With vasectomy reversals, adequate mobilisation of the two ends of the vas is required without devascularising the vas. A simple method to avoid tension at the end on the procedure is described.

Place a 4/0 Vicryl stay suture in the adventitia on each of the cut vasa. At the end of the procedure, tie the stay sutures together and adjust the tension just so that the anastomosis can be seen to be tension free. As the anastomosis heals and the paratesticular tissues adhere to the anastomosis, the final result should be tension free.

118

Intracorporeal perforation during penile implantation

Suks Minhas

Intracorporeal perforation during penile implantation is a relatively common but difficult problem to manage. The key points in trying to avoid this are to anticipate when the situation may arise. In this context, patients who have a fibrotic penis, in particular those who are post priapism, have Peyronie's disease or had a previously infected implant will be at increased risk of perforation.

The key is to try and recognise perforation during implantation. If the dilation is particularly difficult then try and avoid this by ensuring that you have adequate exposure of the area. My normal incision is usually a penile-scrotal incision, but I always warn the patient with a potentially fibrotic penis that we will need to make a further incision circumferentially distally in the case of perforation, or if a difficult dilation is anticipated. When dilating for intracorporeal fibrosis, ensure that your left hand pushes the scissors or dilator towards you, as often there is a tendency during dilation to push the scissors towards the neurovascular bundle and hence perforation can occur.

During the surgery, if a perforation is suspected then ensure that you have the right instruments and appropriate exposure. Distal perforation can be expected if distally the tip of the dilator, such as a Hegar dilator, lies within the glans or placing two dilators down the corpora distally, the two ends meet or cross over. Proximal perforation can be more difficult to diagnose but certainly the same principles apply if there is a discrepancy in the measurement of the dilatators, and when they sit on the pubic bone there is a discrepancy in height of more than 1 cm, then corporeal perforation proximally should be suspected.

In case of distal perforation at the level of the penile shaft, this can be detected by seeing the tip of the dilator protruding superficially. In such cases redilation can be undertaken. If dilation has already been performed and the surgeon is happy that this is adequate on the contralateral side, then place a dilator in the contralateral corpora body. This will aid dilation on the ipsilateral perforated side. Gently dilate with Metzenbaum scissors towards the tip, again making sure that the curve of the scissors is directed laterally. In some instances, it will be difficult to dilate, particularly with a fibrotic penis, and a separate incision will need to be made with a separate corporotomy to ensure that the dilating scissors or dilator is seen more distally.

Proximally the dilation can be more difficult and if perforation is suspected. Redilation can be performed with a dilator on the contralateral side if there is no perforation on that side. Commence dilation by ensuring that you have adequate traction on the penis and this is helped by having a 3.0 Vicryl stay suture within the glans, which is held up by an assistant. The key here is surgical exposure and feel rather than actual direct visualisation of the perforation as you will not see this. The perforated corpora can then be redilated gently opening the scissors towards the pubic bone. Scissors can be directed with the left hand if you are right handed and vice versa, whilst dilation with the scissors in the opposite hand. This is the reason why on difficult implants you should ensure that you have adequate exposure of both penile crura down towards the bulbar urethra as this allows you to directly feel the dilators and the scissors as you are dissecting.

In a distal perforation, particularly if the perforation is through the corporeal tips, an undersized malleable implant can be used which is then sutured with a PDS stitch. I find the Coloplast malleable implant particularly useful in these circumstances and a Vicryl stitch can be placed through the corporotomy and the corpora closed in this manner with interrupted stitches with occasional stitches gathering up the implant's outer surface. This ensures that the penile implant remains in place but of course it can still migrate subsequently. With a more proximal perforation, I do not use a windsock but rather will use a smaller length of prosthesis distally and later come back and perform further surgery and redilate the proximal crura. Alternatively, you can estimate the length of the implant by measurement of the contralateral side (if this has not been perforated!) and then downsize this relative to the length of the crural measurement. Therefore an implant on this side can be placed which is shorter, again sutured in place with Vicryl as the corporotomy is closed. In some instances, this will suffice in itself for sexual function but usually patients will need to come back to theatre for redilation of the area which is subsequently made easier after about 3 months.

During surgery, ensure that you perform a salvage washout to ensure asepsis which, in my experience, reduces the risk of infection in these difficult cases.

PART 6
Female Urology

Top Tips in Urology, Second Edition. Edited by John McLoughlin, Neil Burgess,
Hanif Motiwala, Mark J. Speakman, Andrew Doble and John D. Kelly.
© 2013 John Wiley & Sons, Ltd. Published 2013 by John Wiley & Sons, Ltd.

119

Recurrent cystocoele and rectocoele repair using modified mesh: new technique

Rob Gray and Hanif Motiwala

The prolapse repair has an up to 30% failure rate at any given time in its natural history. The difficult ones are those which are recurrent from the previously failed repair. There is controversy over the use of mesh but it is less controversial to use mesh in a previously failed repair as there is evidence of very high success for its use. There are many commercially available kits on the market for this and costs range from £600 to over £1000.

We have designed a very simple mesh repair avoiding complex needle passages and passes. This is used for both cystocoele and rectocoele for recurrent cases.

After dissecting out cystocoele and rectocoele and reconstructing the anatomical layer again with Vicryl sutures, the repair is strengthened with Parietene Progrip mesh. The mesh is sized up according to the defect. The wings are passed through the endopelvic fascia anteriorly or sacrococcygeal ligament posteriorly. The mesh has a self-sticking ability and this will stay without any need for suturing as the patient will have a 24-h pack. A further few stitches are placed laterally to fix this along the lateral wall. See Figures 119.1–119.5.

Our personal experience over 50 cases has yielded excellent results comparable to the commercially available kits reported in the literature.

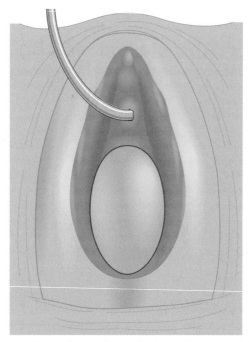

Figure 119.1 This view shows the urethra with the catheter in and the anterior vaginal wall as seen inside a draped area.

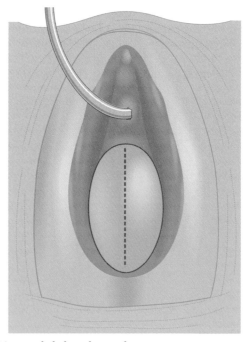

Figure 119.2 Incision made below the urethra.

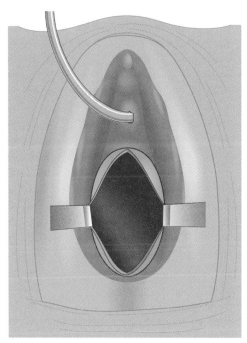

Figure 119.3 Cystocoele dissected out.

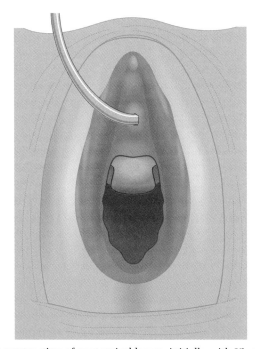

Figure 119.4 Reconstruction of anatomical layers, initially with Vicryl sutures.

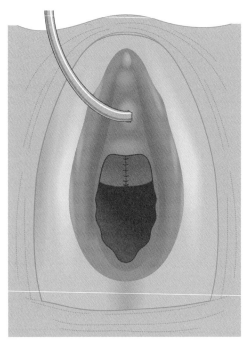

Figure 119.5 Mesh is passed through the endopelvic fascia and sutured into place.

120

Eroded transvaginal tape

Rizwan Hamid

It is a challenge to treat a patient after a failed eroded transvaginal tape. The eroded tape has to be removed but the subsequent management is difficult. After tape removal, the tissues become scarred and fibrotic and hence another synthetic sling is not recommended.

However, after removal of an eroded tape, if a Martius fat pad is inserted at the same time, this not only provides support to the urethral defect but can also provide a good base for subsequent insertion of a synthetic sling rather than an autologous one.

The procedure should be performed as described below (Figure 120.1).

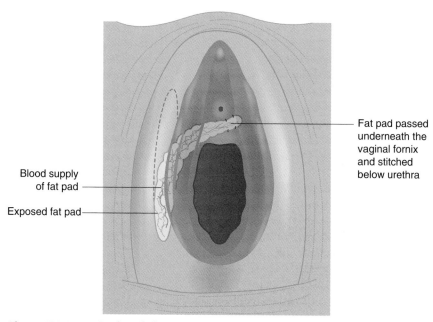

Blood supply of fat pad

Exposed fat pad

Fat pad passed underneath the vaginal fornix and stitched below urethra

Figure 120.1 Repair of eroded transvaginal tape.

After making an inverted U incision in the anterior vaginal wall, the eroded tape is excised as much as possible. The defect in the urethra is closed in two layers over a 12F catheter. A Martius fat pad is then harvested from either of the labia majora. Once a sufficient length is mobilized, it is then tunnelled underneath the vaginal fornix and under the reconstructed urethra. It is stitched in place by four stitches on either side of the urethra. The vaginal incision is closed over the fat pad.

In a small percentage of cases this procedure alone will maintain continence. However, in the remainder a subsequent anti-incontinence procedure will be required. Hence, 3–6 months later, a second synthetic sling can be inserted on top of the Martius fat pad. This is performed via an incision in the anterior vaginal wall and placing the transvaginal tape in a standard way. The tape will pass superficial to the Martius fat pad, with the pad between the urethra and the sling. The tape can be passed through the fat pad and onto the obturator foramen in case of a transobturator tape. The anterior vaginal incision is closed in the standard fashion and the follow-up is the same as for the first tape procedure.

This technique helps to provide an opportunity to safely insert a second synthetic sling in cases where the first sling has eroded. Otherwise, as mentioned above, due to scarring and fibrosis, the only vaginal sling that can be utilised is an autologous sling, with its associated morbidity.

121

Midurethral tension-free tapes

Neil Harris

Synthetic suburethral tapes are the 'gold standard' treatment for stress urinary incontinence (SUI). The majority of patients will undergo urodynamic evaluation prior to surgery, not only to confirm the diagnosis of SUI but to exclude other types of bladder dysfunction which might affect surgical outcome. NICE guidelines, however, suggest that preoperative urodynamics are not required in patients presenting with symptoms of pure stress incontinence. Remember that other types of pelvic floor dysfunction often co-exist. These include pelvic organ prolapse and defaecatory dysfunction.

There are numerous types of tape available, but all are either retropubic (e.g. TVT) or transobturator (TOT). Published data show little difference in outcomes between the two types. Side-effects and perioperative risks are slightly different.

Alternatives to the tapes include colposuspension (rarely indicated nowadays), autologous slings (useful for refractory stress incontinence, especially if intrinsic sphincter weakness is present) and periurethral bulking.

Consent and counselling prior to surgery are essential. Warn patients of the risks of persistent stress incontinence (around 20%), development or worsening of overactive bladder symptoms, tape erosion/extrusion, voiding dysfunction and bladder injury.

Surgery can be done using general or local anaesthesia, although most cases are performed under GA.

Ensure patients are voiding satisfactorily before discharge and check urinary residuals. If residuals are high, patients should be taught self-catheterisation and residuals usually diminish over the next few weeks. If voiding dysfunction persists, the tape has probably been placed too tight and will require division or loosening. Loosening of tapes needs to be done within 2 weeks, otherwise the tape will be 'fixed' as a result of tissue ingrowth and division will be required.

122

Treatment of TVT mesh eroding the bladder

Georgina Wilson

Examine the woman under anaesthesia with careful inspection of the anterior vaginal wall with a Simms speculum to retract the posterior wall of the vagina to exclude concomitant vaginal extrusion of tape.

Carefully examine the urethra with a 0° cystoscope to check there is no TVT mesh in the urethra.

Examine the bladder with a 30° and 70° cystoscope. Most erosions of mesh are found at the 10/11o'clock position of the bladder close to the bladder neck and you may need the 70° cystoscope to visualise it well.

Once the mesh erosion is located, introduce a ureteric catheter through the cystoscope and through this place a 500 μm holmium laser fibre. The ureteric catheter acts to stabilise the laser fibre. Place the laser fibre a few millimetres from the mesh erosion and then stroke the laser fibre over the surface of the eroded mesh (similar to the 'painting' movement used with the laser to destroy ureteric stones). The mesh will spring apart with this movement and the fibres will appear to retract. Continue until no more mesh can be seen.

At the end of the procedure place a urethral catheter and leave for 72 h.

Plan a repeat procedure to check all tape destroyed in 4–6 weeks. Often small fibres of mesh will be found on the second examination and you can treat again with the laser as above.

PART 7
General

Top Tips in Urology, Second Edition. Edited by John McLoughlin, Neil Burgess,
Hanif Motiwala, Mark J. Speakman, Andrew Doble and John D. Kelly.
© 2013 John Wiley & Sons, Ltd. Published 2013 by John Wiley & Sons, Ltd.

123

Circumcision

Andrew Doble

The prepuce is retracted and an incision is made circumferentially around the mucosal aspect of the shaft 2 cm below the coronal sulcus. The difficulty of cutting the penile shaft skin in a straight line is overcome by using sinus forceps. A mark is made on the dorsal aspect of the penile skin at the level of the coronal sulcus and two small clips are applied to the prepuce, one dorsally and one ventrally. The glans penis is depressed and the sinus forceps applied with the tips at the mark on the dorsal aspect and angled so that less prepuce is removed from the ventral aspect of the shaft. An assistant then holds the small clips vertically and a blade cuts the prepuce above the sinus forcep's limbs, thereby protecting the glans (Figure 123.1). Any residual mucosa is removed from the shaft, bipolar diathermy used to achieve haemostasis and mucosal skin apposition achieved with an interrupted 4/0 Vicryl suture.

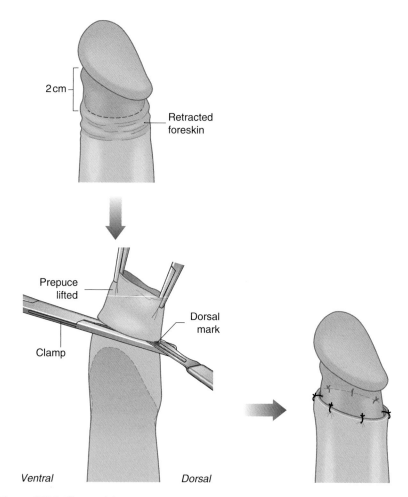

Figure 123.1 Circumcision.

124

Dressing a circumcision

Simon Bott

As a trainee I was shown and tried a number of different dressings to apply to a circumcision, but they all fall off. The best way, I think, is to use a crepe bandage. I apply a non-adhesive dressing such as Jelonet folded 1 cm wide and laid over the incision. I then apply a gauze and then a 2 inch crepe bandage. The crepe bandage applies some slight pressure for haemostasis and also ensures that the dressing does not come off, thereby potentially reducing the risk of infection. I ask the patients to remove the dressing after 48 h.

125

Postcircumcision dressing: the gauze sporran

Andrew Doble

After completing the surgery and applying Vaseline or petroleum jelly to the suture line and glans, dressings often pose problems. A dry gauze dressing with a hole creates a suitable covering and a means of collecting any small amounts of blood loss from the wound (Figure 125.1).

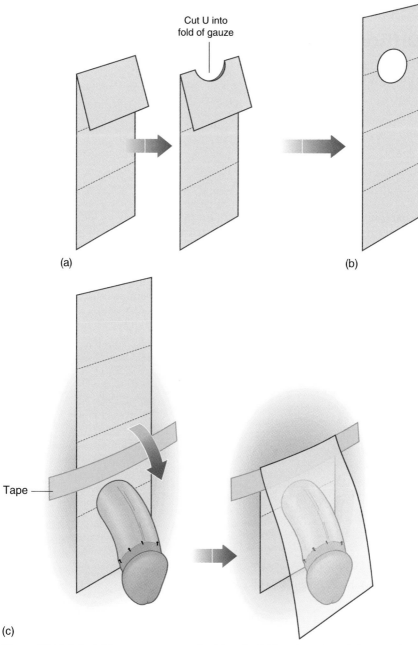

Figure 125.1 (a,b,c) The gauze sporran. Position the fold and cutting of the U to the size of the penis, so that there is gauze underneath the penile shaft as well as covering once the flap has been folded down.

126

Difficult reduction of paraphimosis

Andrew Doble

A paraphimosis that has been present for over 48 h may be difficult to reduce due to the oedema created by the constricting ring. Instillation of 2–5 mL of 1% lignocaine with an orange needle into the constricting ring will allow incision of the ring transversely (Figure 126.1), thereby reducing the constriction and facilitating reduction of the paraphimosis. No sutures are required as the wound will be on the mucosal aspect of the prepuce once reduced.

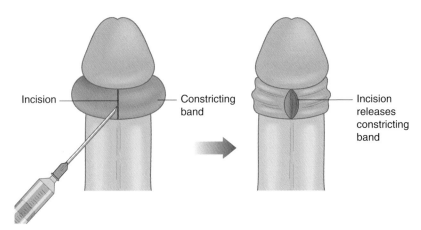

Figure 126.1 Reduction of difficult paraphimosis.

127

Round-bodied needles

Richard Bell

Use a round-bodied Vicryl Rapide for circumcisions and scrotal skin as it completely avoids bleeding from the suture puncture sites.

128

Bladder clots

Ling Lee

Sucking small clots via a flexible cystoscope

Place the end of the flexiscope over the clot. Undo the water connection to the scope and suck the clot with a 10 mL syringe (Figure 128.1). This directed suction is very effective at clearing small clots.

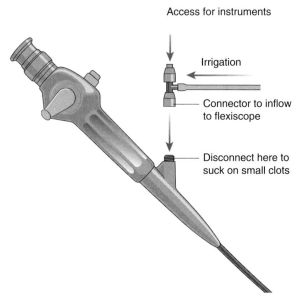

Access for instruments

Irrigation

Connector to inflow to flexiscope

Disconnect here to suck on small clots

Figure 128.1 Flexible cystoscope inflow tap removed to allow access for clot suction.

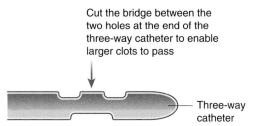

Cut the bridge between the
two holes at the end of the
three-way catheter to enable
larger clots to pass

Three-way
catheter

Figure 128.2 Hole at catheter tip enlarged to facilitate evacuation of large clots.

Larger clots in the bladder

For large clots in the bladder, I enlarge the hole at the end of a three-way catheter to facilitate the drawing out of clots. Some catheter balloons may be breached so you will need to use a new one if it has to stay in (Figure 128.2).

129

Performing a flexible cystoscopy for a bladder which is full of debris

Asif Muneer

On occasion, the urologist is presented with a patient who requires a diagnostic flexible cystoscopy due to a single episode of haematuria, suspected bladder stones or suspected foreign bodies such as remnants of the catheter/catheter balloon. Generally these patients tend to be elderly with multiple co-morbidities and are often confused.

If the bladder is full of phosphate debris which makes the views suboptimal, rather than repeat washouts of the bladder which often fail to completely optimise the view, one can perform an 'air cystoscopy'.

Empty the bladder first using a catheter and then use a bladder syringe to fill the bladder with approximately 200 mL of air. Then insert the flexible cystoscope. For female patients, irrigating fluid is not usually required due to the short urethra. In men, gentle irrigation can be used to negotiate the urethra. You will find that the debris is no longer floating in the bladder and impairing the view but has sunk to the posterior wall. Perform a routine cystoscopy and then gently open the irrigation to flush away the debris to ensure that the posterior wall is free of any lesion.

130

Passing a urethra catheter across a stricture after a guidewire is passed via the flexible cystoscope

Ling Lee

Using a small no. 15 blade, make a small oblique cut to expose the central lumen (Figure 130.1). This makes it easier to push through the stricture and over the guidewire in the bladder. It works with a Sympa-Cath as it doesn't breach the balloon mechanism. Splitting the end of the catheter to allow a guidewire to pass also works but I find it less successful. This also makes subsequent change of catheter over a guidewire easier.

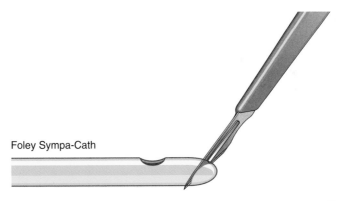

Foley Sympa-Cath

Figure 130.1 Cutting the tip of the catheter obliquely to expose the central lumen.

131

Inserting a catheter over a guidewire

Simon Bott

In difficult catheterisation it is sometimes necessary to insert a guidewire up the urethra into the bladder under vision and then insert a catheter over the guidewire. If an open-ended catheter is not available, rather than remove the tip of a standard Foley catheter I pass an orange Venflon through the tip of the catheter via one of the eyes at the tip. The distal end of the wire can then be placed through the orange Venflon and brought out through the eye of the catheter. The Venflon can then be removed and the tip of the wire fed back through the eye and up the catheter. Some lubricating jelly placed down the catheter will facilitate this. The catheter can then be passed over the wire, ensuring that the wire is kept taut. Once in the bladder, the wire can be easily withdrawn.

132

Cryoanalgesia for prostate biopsy

Simon Robinson and Hanif Motiwala

Transrectal ultrasound and biopsy can still be a painful procedure. We describe a simple, additional, complication-free method for reducing pain during biopsies by cooling the rectal surface with a condom containing ice (Figure 132.1). We have looked at this prospectively using a visual analogue score.

Two minutes before the local anaesthetic injection and biopsy, 5 cc of ice is inserted into the rectum via a condom. The water is placed within the condom using a syringe, the condom is placed flat in the freezer and the water forms a smooth convex surface, to enable gentle insertion to the rectum.

The two pictures in Figure 132.2 are examples of how cryoanalgesia diminishes nerve conduction and sensation.

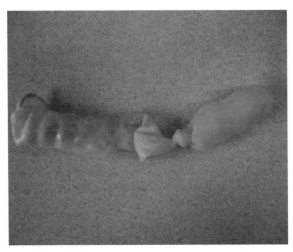

Figure 132.1 Ice-filled condom.

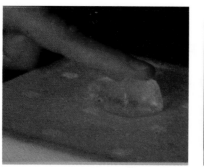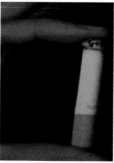

Figure 132.2 Contact between ice cube and finger can lead to reduced sensation.

Pain experienced with lidocaine alone yields a score of nearly 3/10 and this is almost halved when cryoanalgesia is added. This simple modification of analgesia adds little time and allows a significant reduction in pain experience.

133

Pain relief in epididymo-orchitis

Andrew Doble

Local anaesthetic (10 mL 1% lignocaine or 5 mL 1% lignocaine and 5 mL 0.5% bupivicaine mixed together) injected into the spermatic cord at the neck of the scrotum will provide instant relief and permit the application of adequate scrotal support. Subsequent pain control will be facilitated.

134

Hydrocoele

Senthil Nathan

After resecting the sac when opening the parietal tunica vaginalis, one should use a no. 15 or 11 blade knife. The knife should be stabbed into the hydrocoele sac and held in position at 45°. The hydrocoele fluid will run along the lower border of the knife and neatly drain into a kidney dish. This will avoid splashing fluid all over the place during the procedure.

135

Epididymal cyst

Senthil Nathan

When trying to enucleate an epididymal cyst completely, one must use a no. 15 blade knife to cut open the visceral layer of the tunica vaginalis. Lying just under the visceral layer will be the plane at which to dissect the cyst completely without causing damage to the nearby vessels and nerves.

136

Shape of the male urethra

Simon Bott

The male urethra in the flaccid state is S shaped. When inserting a catheter, the penis is pulled up 90° to the anterior abdominal wall and this straightens out the first curve in the urethra, but there is still a second curve at the bulbar urethra. We are frequently called by colleagues to be told that the catheter cannot be passed as it is getting 'stuck in the prostate'. However, almost invariably this is because the catheter has made a false passage in the bulbar urethra rather than 'going round the bend'. To straighten the second curve after the catheter has been introduced down the full length of the penile urethra, the penis should be pulled down between the legs. Whilst this does not completely remove the bend, it does straighten it and facilitate catheter passage into the bladder. This should reduce the risk of developing false passages and failed catheterisation.

137

Local anaesthetic injection through skin

Paul McInerney

One nuisance of local anaesthetic injection is bleeding from the injection site. I have found this can be minimised by retaining a little bit of the local in the syringe prior to withdrawing the needle, and as the needle is withdrawn through the skin margin, the remaining local is injected at the exit site to raise a little bleb and tamponade any bleeding at the site. It doesn't work particularly well with a large-bore green needle because the exit aperture is too wide and it tends to spray around, but it is much more successful with smaller bore needles such as blue or orange ones.

138

Transrectal ultrasound

John McLoughlin

There are a number of simple things that can make life easier for the patient and operator.

Correct positioning

The patient needs to lie slightly off centre in the left lateral position, i.e. rolled with their torso slightly away from the operator. The tendency is for patients to talk and/or roll backwards which makes scanning the right side awkward (when the probe handle is angled down towards the bed).

Digital rectal examination

When performing digital rectal examination (DRE), leave your finger in for 15–20 sec if the patient is 'gripping' your finger. This will help them relax their sphincter. If they still grip then push your index finger laterally out against the sphincter in 3, 6, 9 and 12 o'clock positions to further relax it. Remember, patients who grip are more prone to collapse on you afterwards.

If you are using a B-K probe, which has a notch that can make it uncomfortable to insert, push the side of the probe without the notch backwards against the anal sphincter as you insert it so that the actual notch is pulled away, making less contact on the opposite side.

Avoid movements that rotate and swivel the probe around (corkscrew type movements) as these are uncomfortable for patients.

The needle

The bevel of the needle should be orientated so that the sharp apex as opposed to the flat portion makes contact with the rectal wall (Figure 138.1). This ensures a quick puncture, less pain, less tearing of the rectal wall as it doesn't slip along the mucosa and also helps you determine the correct plane to start infiltration. The easiest way to do this is to always set your needle on the

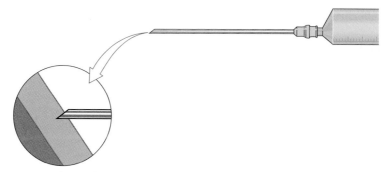

Figure 138.1 The angle of entry of the anaesthetic needle onto the rectal wall is very important.

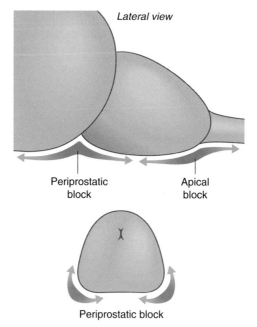

Figure 138.2 Direction of movement of anaesthetic along periprostatic tissue planes.

syringe in the same way, so that by looking at the offset on the syringe, you know which way up your needle is.

Demonstrate a blank fire of the needle gun to the patient as the noise often makes them jump initially.

Local anaesthetic

I use 20 mL 0.5% marcain and place it as an apical midline plus bilateral periprostatic blocks (Figure 138.2). You really want to see the local anaesthetic tracking under and alongside the gland to ensure good results. Laterally, I infiltrate as far back as the base of the seminal vesicles along to the tip of the apex.

Getting the best cores

The core length or calibre can be better from one side of the prostate compared to the other. This can be corrected by rotating the needle gun around on its axis so the needle fires from the opposite side of the firing chamber.

Bleeding

It is possible to hit sizeable rectal wall arteries with your biopsy needle. The result can be heavy rectal bleeding. Place a very well-lubricated small 10×10 cm gauze swab around your gloved extended index finger and perform a DRE, pushing the rectal wall anterolaterally, and in doing so compressing the wall of the rectum against one of the lateral lobes.

139

Modified transrectal biopsy of prostate

Ruzi Begum, Rob Gray and Hanif Motiwala

When faced with the prospect of having to do a biopsy on the ward or in the outpatient setting in the absence of transrectal ultrasound guidance, a useful trick is to use the sheath supplied with a 21G spinal needle (ask your friendly anaesthetist for one!). In advanced prostate cancer, one or two simple biopsies are all that is needed.

The spinal needle comes with a sheath (Figure 139.1) which will work as a guiding sheath. If secured to the index finger (Figure 139.2), one can then run the biopsy needle up and down the sheath safely, in a sterile fashion and avoid a nasty sharps injury!

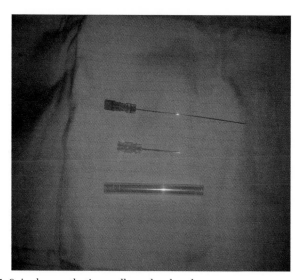

Figure 139.1 Spinal anaesthetic needle and a sheath.

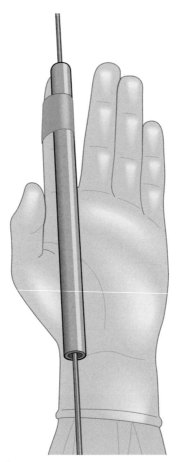

Figure 139.2 Sheath in action.

140

Transperineal biopsy probe set-up

John McLoughlin

Here is a simple way to stop the endocavity balloon slipping around the probe when performing transperineal template biopsies (it can even fall off the probe when you inflate the balloon for the first time which is a real pain). Wrap a length of 1 inch Transpore tape on the end of the balloon and onto the probe (Figure 140.1). The probe needs to be really dry and have neither lubricant nor ultrasonic gel as otherwise it will not stick.

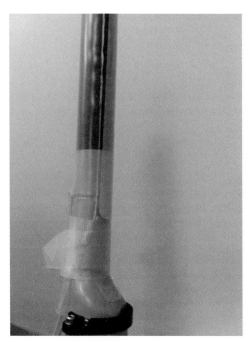

Figure 140.1 Tape wrapped around end of endocavity balloon.

141

Changing a difficult or encrusted suprapubic catheter

John McLoughlin

I have found this useful for obese female patients with a blocked or heavily encrusted catheter that doesn't budge when pulled prior to changing it. I have, on occasion, also done this for the morbidly obese patient with a contracted bladder (the clue being that they may well have needed an open suprapubic insertion in the first place) where there is a chance that the tract may be lost easily.

- Clean the suprapubic skin area and lubricate the portion of the catheter that lies externally with sterile Instillagel.
- Insert a flexible cystoscope via urethra and using a rat tooth forceps, pull the tip of the catheter into the urethra and out into the outside world between the legs. Because encrustation occurs inside the bladder, this works well as the outer portion is free of build-up.
- Cut the tip of the catheter off above the balloon and then pull the catheter back along the suprapubic tract and out and quickly replace the suprapubic catheter down the tract.

If there is real concern that the tract may be lost during attempted catheter exchange then:

- place a long length of 2/0 Prolene suture through the cut end of the catheter as it sits there out of the urethra and tie a knot, before withdrawing back along the tract. The suture length has to be long enough to protrude out of both the urethra and the suprapubic site at the same time
- pull back the catheter and, once both catheter and suture are out of the suprapubic wound, cut the suture
- insert the suture through the eye of the new catheter that is to be inserted along the tract and tie a knot
- relubricate the catheter. Pull the urethral end of the suture and the catheter will follow. Pull it until the catheter tip extrudes out of the urethra and then cut the suture
- finally pull back the suprapubic catheter to relocate the catheter tip just inside the bladder and reinflate the balloon.

The procedure takes about 2–3 min.

If all else fails and you have lost the tract already, insert a flexible cystoscope down the tract and use a Sensor guidewire to find your way back into the bladder.

142

How to predict the difficult catheter? Use the force!

K. Mozolowski and John G. Calleary

Urethral catheterisation/flexible cystoscopy requires the instillation of lubricating or local anaesthetic gel solutions. The rate of instillation of the gel is directly associated with urethral pain experienced due to distension. Distension is limited by urethral pathology such as stricture disease and in some cases by occlusive prostatic disease.

We have noticed that when anything other than gentle depression of the plunger is required, there is a greater likelihood of difficulty in insertion of a catheter or flexible cystoscope. After standard preparation, the most important step is to empty any air bubble(s) from the syringe by gentle pressure on the plunger in an inverted syringe. The gel should move easily on gentle pressure. Then the same gentle pressure is used to insert the gel. If resistance is felt or the gel appears to exude from the urethra, the catheterisation can be difficult. This is most noticeable in urethral strictures.

143

Urodynamics

Sarah Wood

In some patients it is not possible to measure abdominal pressure (Pabd) using a rectal line. For example, if the rectal line is constantly expelled due to high rectal pressures, if there is rectal prolapse or after abdomino-perineal (AP) resection if it is not possible to use the ileal conduit. In this situation is it possible to use a nasogastric route instead. Oesophageal manometry catheters are available. By passing the catheter 55 cm from the nares, the distal 10 cm should lie within the stomach and provide equivalent abdominal pressures to rectal lines when the patient is lying (small adjustments may be needed when sitting or standing). By passing 20 mL saline down the catheter and listening with a stethoscope, it is possible to confirm position in the stomach.

PART 8
Clinical Management

Top Tips in Urology, Second Edition. Edited by John McLoughlin, Neil Burgess, Hanif Motiwala, Mark J. Speakman, Andrew Doble and John D. Kelly.
© 2013 John Wiley & Sons, Ltd. Published 2013 by John Wiley & Sons, Ltd.

144

Neurourology

Philip van Kerrebroeck

Every functional problem of the lower urinary tract must be considered as potentially of neurological origin until the contrary has been proven and every urologist should be able to perform a basic neurourological examination. Psychosomatic causes for lower urinary tract dysfunction are a diagnosis of exclusion but a neurological disease and psychosomatic problems can co-exist.

The main aims of therapy in neurourology are preservation of kidney function and quality of life for the patient. Both these goals have to be balanced against each other in the short term but also in the medium and long term, which can mean that a compromise between these two may be necessary at some point.

In order to achieve maximum preservation of kidney function, intravesical pressure has to be kept as low as possible (compliance <20 and pressure <40 cmH_2O). A slow-fill urodynamic investigation is necessary to plan the therapeutic approach in order to balance both storage and voiding function.

Kidney function in patients with severe motor problems and low muscular mass can only be estimated with a creatinine clearance, as serum creatinine will remain low, even if renal insufficiency is developing.

If spontaneous micturition is not possible at low pressure, evacuation of urine is preferably done by clean intermittent (self) catheterisation. Other methods (e.g. Valsalva, Credé) will risk complications (vesicoureteral reflux, prolapse, haemorrhoids). The optimal frequency of catheterisation in order to minimise the number of urinary tract infections is between minimum 4 and maximum 6 per 24 h.

Ultrasound of the kidneys at least once a year is indicated, and more frequently in cases with complications, e.g. infection.

145

Managing urinary tract damage due to ketamine abuse

Dan Wood

Ketamine is well known as a safe and effective anaesthetic and analgesic, and it remains so under appropriate medical supervision. Over the last few years urologists have begun to recognise a syndrome of severe lower urinary tract symptoms in people who have persistently used ketamine as a recreational drug. Initial case reports have given way to larger series and the recognition of a growing problem. The clinical syndrome includes a very small, painful bladder, incontinence, upper tract obstruction, papillary necrosis and hepatic dysfunction.

There appears to be both a time- and a dose-dependent relationship – both with the onset and the improvement of symptoms. Clinicians encountering patients with the above syndrome need to ask about the use of recreational drugs in order to establish a diagnosis. Initial assessment needs to eliminate a urinary tract infection; with a midstream urine (MSU), a computed tomography (CT) urogram is important to rule out upper tract strictures and cystoscopy is needed to assess baseline capacity. Initial management is supportive with chronic pain support. The pain is such that many patients can only achieve adequate pain relief by continuing the ketamine. With good drug agency support and a combination of buprenorphine patches, co-codamol and amitriptyline, adequate analgesia and rehabilitation are achievable.

Once a patient has stopped their ketamine use, assuming there is no urgent need to intervene (i.e. upper tract obstruction), both clinician and patient should aim to wait as long as possible before surgical intervention as extirpative surgery and reconstruction is a major undertaking, requiring detailed patient counselling and preparation, and may be avoidable.

146

Top tips for foreskin assessment

Dan Wood

The title of this section is deliberately chosen. In the past many surgeons have performed circumcision with 'soft' indications. The natural history of the foreskin begins with a physiological phimosis that resolves in the majority by 10 years and 95% by age 16 years. In a statement from the British Association of Paediatric Urologists, they note a decrease in circumcision rates from 30,000 to 20,000 over a period of 10 years to 2007.

The only absolute indication for circumcision is a scarred foreskin as a result of balanitis xerotica obliterans (BXO). Relative indications are recurrent inflammation or balanitis – the history for these needs to be examined carefully as mild intermittent redness is not a concern whereas pain, discharge or bleeding should be regarded more seriously. The additional, relative indication is the presence of anatomical abnormalities in the urinary tract as a means of preventing urinary tract infection.

In distinguishing normal from abnormal, the examining doctor needs to know that ballooning, preputial pearls and flowering/ballooning of the foreskin are normal. A scarred ring of white tissue that prevents retraction is indicative of BXO and patients with this should be offered circumcision.

Many patients and their parents attend clinic with the preconception that the path to circumcision is a formality. This is an out-of-date view. Medical indications for circumcision are rare in all ages – reassurance and explanation of this take time (sometimes longer that it would take to perform the operation!) but are vital. Circumcision can result in complications in up to 7% of patients and in those who need something, topical steroids and preputioplasty will resolve the clinical problem for the majority.

147

Lower urinary tract symptom progression

Mark J. Speakman

Most patients with lower urinary tract symptoms (LUTS) who have problems (most easily assessed on the quality of life question 8 on the International Prostate Symptom Score [IPSS]) simply require treatment with an alpha-blocker after minimal investigation. Ten to 20% of patients will have a significant storage component and they can benefit from the addition of a modern anticholinergic drug provided they do not have a large residual volume (>200 mL).

Some patients, however, have more significant disease. The risk of progression of symptoms, the need for surgery or the possibility of retention is predictable in many if properly considered at initial and subsequent assessment. If a patient has more than two risk factors for progression, the addition of a 5-alpha reductase inhibitor makes clinical and commercial sense.

These risk factors include:

- symptoms (IPSS >13/35)
- increasing symptom severity at review
- poor symptom response to initial medical therapy
- bother (>3/5)
- flow rate (<10 mL/sec)
- age (>70 years)
- prostatic volume (>40 cc)
- prostate-specific antigen (PSA) (>1.4 ng/mL)
- residual volume (?? >200 mL)
- inflammation (presence on needle biopsy).

The relative risk reduction of progression of approximately 55–65% with drugs like dutasteride or finasteride is likely to be achieved in all patients but cost-effectiveness is only achieved in those with a significant risk. It should not be difficult to differentiate between the 55 year old with the small prostate with a low PSA and a reasonable flow, etc., and the 75 year old with a large prostate, a PSA of 2.2, severe symptoms, etc.

It should not be forgotten, however, that surgery remains the most effective treatment for true bladder outlet obstruction.

148

Management of chronic prostatitis/chronic pelvic pain syndrome: top 10 tips

J. Curtis Nickel

1. Chronic prostate infection (category II chronic bacterial prostatitis) can be ruled out by performing a pre and post massage test

Comparing the culture results of the initial urine specimen (first 10 cc) after a vigorous prostate massage to a traditional midstream urine (MSU) taken before the massage is as accurate for diagnosing chronic prostate infection as the traditional 4-glass Meares-Stamey test in more than 95% of patients. This is most effective before antibiotics have been prescribed but can be successful by waiting for a period of time after antibiotic therapy has been completed. The test is positive if the post-massage test cultures any uropathogenic bacteria when the pre-massage specimen is sterile or when the post-massage test cultures at least one log more bacteria than in the pre-massage culture. A diagnosis of chronic prostate infection allows the physician to prescribe long-term antimicrobial therapy (at least 4–6 weeks).

2. There is no clinical rationale to perform microscopic evaluation of prostate-specific specimens in clinical practice

Textbooks and review articles on non-bacterial prostatitis will differentiate cases based on the presence or absence of white blood cells seen on microscopy in the differential urine or expressed prostatic secretion specimens. To date, there is no evidence to prescribe different treatments based on the differentiation of the inflammatory category of chronic prostatitis/chronic pelvic pain syndrome (CP/CPPS) (category IIIA) from the non-inflammatory (category IIIB). In fact, asymptomatic men without prostatitis-like symptoms also have white blood cells in their expressed prostatic secretions and post-massage urine specimens.

3. The NIH Chronic Prostatitis Symptom Index (NIH-CPSI) saves time and frustration in clinical practice

The NIH-CPSI, a 9-question index, explores the most important domains of a patient's experience and can be completed by the patient in 5 min. A quick review of the completed form allows the physician to determine the location, frequency and severity of the pain, the voiding and storage symptoms, and the impact of the condition on the patient's activities and quality of life. It streamlines the initial history of present illness. The total score is used to assess progress over time. A 25% (or 6-point) decrease in symptom score should be regarded as a realistic successful outcome.

4. Learn the phenotypic approach to CPPS classification employing UPOINT

Chronic pelvic pain syndrome is not a homogeneous condition. Although all patients have pelvic-related pain and many have voiding and sexual dysfunction, they arrive by many different aetiological and pathogenic pathways. UPOINT indentifies the six main clinical phenotypes that can be diagnosed using standard clinical evaluation. These phenotypes include Urinary (storage and/or voiding symptoms), Psychosocial (depression, maladaptive coping, poor social support), Organ specific (major pain site or generator is the prostate – typical pain and symptoms identified with light to normal prostate palpation), Infection (organisms identified in post-massage specimen or remote history of urinary tract infection or previous response to antibiotics), Neurological/Systemic (neuropathic pain syndrome or associated syndrome such as irritable bowel syndrome or fibromyalgia), and Tenderness of pelvic muscles (pelvic floor dysfunction or pelvic floor myofascial pain).

5. Develop individual treatment plans for each patient by focusing therapies on specific UPOINT domains

Therapy should be directed towards each of the phenotypes identified in individual patients. For example, alpha-blockers for U, amitriptyline or counselling for P, quercetin or Cernilton for O, antibiotics for I, gabapentinoids for N and physiotherapy for T.

6. Consider a combination of the 5 as for initial therapy for category III CPPS: Avoidance, Antibiotics, Alpha-blockers, Anti-inflammatories, 5-Alpha reductase inhibitors

Antibiotics can be suggested (weak evidence) in antibiotic-naive men recently diagnosed, even when cultures are negative, or those identified with UPOINT I. However, if patients do not respond, further antibiotic therapy is not indicated.

Alpha-blockers may benefit men with UPOINT U. Anti-inflammatory agents may help men with UPOINT O. 5-Alpha reductase inhibitors may benefit men with UPOINT U or O, particularly those men over 45 with enlarged prostates and lower urinary tract symptoms. However, be warned that monotherapy with these agents (or any single therapy) is going to be doomed to failure in the majority of patients.

7. Multimodal therapy works better than monotherapy

Patients almost always have more than one phenotype and monotherapies directed towards a single problem are unlikely to significantly ameliorate the entire symptom complex. Rational use of multiple concurrent therapies, based on clinical phenotypes, has the best chance of achieving therapeutic goals.

8. Don't disregard the phytotherapies

Evidence from randomised controlled trials has indicated that the herbal therapies quercetin, pollen extracts (Cernilton) and possibly saw palmetto extracts have shown more efficacy than placebo. There are almost no side-effects and, except for cost, there are few downsides in considering these therapies.

9. Get your non-urological colleagues involved

Pain physicians, psychologists, physiotherapists and practitioners of complementary medicine may be able to help your patients when you cannot. A multidisciplinary approach to the management of what eventually becomes a chronic neuropathic pain state with generalised pelvic neuromuscular dysfunction may provide the best symptom amelioration.

10. Set realistic expectations

The best researchers in the world do not know the cause of category III CPPS and the best clinicians cannot offer a complete cure. It is, however, a condition that can be managed and unlike many other chronic and inflammatory pain conditions, can spontaneously resolve ('burn out') over time. The patient must understand that the role of the urologist is to ameliorate symptoms, decrease the impact of the condition and improve quality of life, not necessarily to provide a cure.

149

Uro-gynae tips

Glyn Constantine

The fact that a patient has a finding such as a prolapse or various bladder symptoms doesn't necessarily mean that something needs to be done about it. We should always remember that we can create problems as well as solve them and if there wasn't much of a problem there in the first place, this is not a good situation for the patient. Surgically, when dealing with a prolapse involving the uterus, always give serious consideration to vault support which can prevent many more complex problems arising subsequently.

150

Psychological problems and surgery

Paul McInerney

Surgery does not cure psychological problems and one of the hardest things to do in medicine is nothing. However, it is often the correct approach.

151

Use of analogies to assist with explanation of urological problems

David Nicol

One of the key skills in urology, as with all areas of medical practice, is the ability to communicate with patients. It is critical to use language and terminology that patients can readily comprehend. Medical jargon should be avoided where possible as this may not be understood by patients, who may be reluctant to acknowledge this. Disease processes are often difficult for patients to comprehend, as are the various treatments recommended. In many instances, simple analogies can be used to describe symptoms and explain the rationale behind different management options. Whilst there are numerous examples that may be used and individuals may easily develop their own, I have found a number to be helpful that are illustrative of the principle.

Chronic pain syndromes

These can be frustrating for patients who will often seek multiple opinions as explanations provided do not sufficiently reassure them regarding their symptom complex for which there is ultimately no satisfactory experience. Typical examples in urology include chronic orchalgia and loin pain. In discussing their situation, it can be useful to relate it to other pain problems with which they may be familiar. Headaches and migraines can be used for illustrative purposes. The explanation briefly encompasses a description of headaches and how stress and tiredness may provoke symptoms in the absence of a medical problem. This can be extended to how in selected or severe cases investigations may be undertaken to exclude major problems, including hypertension and intracerebral lesions which may require treatment. Patients will understand from experience that in the overwhelming majority of cases, no treatable cause will be identified and that the patient is left with no option but symptomatic management. This, in some but obviously not all cases, will help them accept that with conditions such as orchalgia, after medical assessment to exclude major pathology or correctable causes, specific intervention beyond symptom control may not be an option.

Surgical intervention for symptomatic conditions

Patients presenting with various symptoms may seek advice as to whether or not they should undergo a surgical option and what is the point at which this should be considered. Surgery for benign prostatic hypertrophy is an example. To help understand the concepts of absolute indications and also the timing of surgery for symptoms, an easy analogy is hip replacement and the various scenarios in which this may be considered. Comparing a fractured hip to the problems of urinary retention or other medical complications of bladder outflow obstruction enables patients to realise that there are circumstances where surgery may be definitely indicated. For even the lay person, the parallel between the obvious need for hip replacement and the need for transurethral resection of prostate (TURP) is then easy to understand as an absolute or highly recommended indication. Similarly, by discussing the timing of joint replacement for arthritis alone it is relatively easy for patients to understand that this depends on how much pain (i.e. symptoms) they are experiencing and the degree to which it affects their quality of life. This leads to a conclusion of the discussion as to the need for and timing of TURP for voiding symptoms in the absence of medical indications.

Pelviureteric junction obstruction

It may be difficult to explain peristasis, bolus and functional obstruction relevant to pelviureteric obstruction. Some patients may find this easier to grasp if the collecting system and ureter are likened to a snake's mouth and body. The relevance of this analogy is that it is easy for someone to imagine a snake swallowing an egg – perhaps using a cartoon-like illustration. Functional obstruction can then be conceptualised as a snake with a loose ring around its neck – it can still eat very small eggs but larger eggs will not pass (or a large soft egg that is squeezed through very slowly). The conversation can move to pyeloplasty or continues with the snake analogy if endopyelotomy is to be undertaken (simply translating to breaking the ring).

Hormone therapy for prostate cancer

The rationale and mechanism of action of androgen deprivation on prostate cancer may be difficult to understand. One simple explanation is to liken androgens for prostate cancer to water for a lawn. If the lawn is not watered regularly it withers but will regrow if watering is resumed. With extended periods of time without regular water, the grass gradually becomes replaced by hardy weeds that require little or no direct watering and that once established are virtually impossible to eradicate …

Using these concepts, numerous other examples can be developed to match almost all clinical scenarios in urology. Obviously, the analogy should not confuse the patient and should be carefully introduced such that its purpose is clear to the patient. Judgement is needed as to the situation in which they may be applicable or necessary – which generally should be only when patients do not appear to understand or accept simple lay explanations (i.e. avoiding medical terminology or jargon including, most importantly, acronyms). It is also important to ensure that their use is not condescending as some, particularly highly educated, patients may take offence at overly simplistic explanations.

Quotes submitted on the back of other tips

Below is a short series of nuggets extracted from covering letters attached to submissions. Some are used to educate, others to motivate.

- It will be all right in the end. If it is not yet all right – it is not yet the end.
- Hope for the best. Plan for the worst. Learn to accept with good grace whatever comes round that corner.
- It is not the first surgical error that kills the patient. It is usually the second error or the consequences of a badly planned approach to correcting the first error that ultimately proves fatal.
- Complications are like a Swiss cheese with lots of holes. Individually they are containable. When they all line up together they prove disastrous.
- You can teach a monkey to operate in a relatively short time but it takes a lifetime to learn to deal objectively with one's own complications.
- I tell my trainees to 'Stand on the shoulders of giants – not in their shadows'.
- You should set yourself goals on a regular basis. When working towards a goal, you will take the knocks on the chin, learn from them and then move on ('what doesn't kill you makes you stronger', to coin the phrase). If you are not working towards a goal you will feel those same setbacks much more and may give up the pursuit altogether. This applies for anything from learning a new procedure to establishing a business case – or even developing a urology service!
- I have a passage written and framed in my office to motivate. It reads 'True champions never surrender. It is one thing to hide psychological frailty; quite another to eliminate it. You need reserves of self-belief that mere mortals find hard to comprehend. Never accept on the basis of probabilities that you are beaten'. No, I haven't been investigated by the GMC!
- If you aim at nothing you will hit it every time.
- When you are getting poor results, ask yourself 'Is it the singer or the song? Is it the surgeon or the operation?'. Take time to reflect before others do it for you! Be honest with yourself without beating yourself up. Be reflective. You should be self-motivated and hard-working. If you are all of the above you have probably already made the grade.

Top Tips in Urology, Second Edition. Edited by John McLoughlin, Neil Burgess, Hanif Motiwala, Mark J. Speakman, Andrew Doble and John D. Kelly.
© 2013 John Wiley & Sons, Ltd. Published 2013 by John Wiley & Sons, Ltd.

Index

Note: page numbers in *italics* refer to figures

Top Tips in Urology, Second Edition. Edited by John McLoughlin, Neil Burgess,
Hanif Motiwala, Mark J. Speakman, Andrew Doble and John D. Kelly.
© 2013 John Wiley & Sons, Ltd. Published 2013 by John Wiley & Sons, Ltd.